FACIAL RECONSTRUCTION WITH LOCAL AND REGIONAL FLAPS

The American Academy of Facial Plastic and Reconstructive Surgery

Series Editor: James D. Smith, M.D.

FACIAL RECONSTRUCTION WITH LOCAL AND REGIONAL FLAPS

Ferdinand F. Becker, M.D., F.A.C.S.
President, Head and Neck
  Surgical Associates
President, Plastic Surgery Center,
  Inc.
Vero Beach, Florida

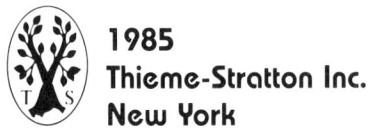

1985
Thieme-Stratton Inc.
New York

Georg Thieme Verlag
Stuttgart ● New York

Thieme-Stratton Inc.
381 Park Avenue South
New York, New York 10016

Series sponsored by the educational committee of The American Academy of Facial Plastic and Reconstructive Surgery

Library of Congress Cataloging in Publication Data

Becker, Ferdinand F.
  Facial reconstruction with local and regional flaps.

  "The American Academy of facial Plastic and Reconstructive Surgery."
  Includes bibliographies and index.
  1. Face—Surgery. 2. Flaps (Surgery) 3. Surgery, Plastic. I. Title. [DNLM: 1. Face—surgery.
2. Surgery, Plastic. 3. Surgical Flaps. WE 705 B388f]
  RD523.B387 1985   617'.52   85-10050
  ISBN 0-86577-199-5 (v. 2)

Cover design by M. Losaw

Printed in the United States of America

FACIAL RECONSTRUCTION WITH LOCAL AND REGIONAL FLAPS
Becker

0-86577-199-5 (Thieme-Stratton Inc.)
3-13-681701-X (Georg Thieme Verlag)

0-86577-137-5 (series)
3-13-656501-0 (series)

Copyright © 1985 by Thieme-Stratton Inc. All rights reserved. No part of this publication may be reused or republished without the express written consent of the publisher.

5 4 3 2 1

Contents

Introduction

1.	Classifications of Facial Flaps	1
2.	Nasolabial Flaps	9
3.	Cheek Flaps and Cervicofacial Flaps	21
4.	Glabellar Flaps and Dorsal Nasal Flaps	37
5.	Rhombic Flaps	45
6.	Bilobed Flaps	55
7.	Lip Flaps	61
8.	Eyelid Reconstruction	79
9.	Forehead Flaps	95
10.	Facial Reconstruction with Multiple Flaps	107
11.	Complications of Facial Flaps	127

Index 157

Dedication

This book is dedicated to my mother, Adeline Moreton Becker, and my father, Ferdinand Francis Becker, II. Without their constant loving support and encouragement my career in this field and this book would not have been possible.

Acknowledgments

My interest in this work has been an evolutionary process and I would like to thank some of the surgeons and teachers who have been most instrumental in developing and directing my interest in this field. My earliest surgical training was in general surgery and later in otolaryngology/head and neck surgery. Dr. Harold G. Tabb of New Orleans, my chief, was instrumental in developing my interests in the extirpation of major tumors of the head, neck and face and encouraged me in learning more about reconstructing the resulting defects. Dr. John Conley of New York had a significant influence in developing my interest in major facial reconstruction and has given me valuable advice, friendship, and encouragement along the way. Dr. Fredric Mohs of Madison, Wisconsin was kind enough to allow me to study under him for a short time and learn his technique of microscopically controlled excision of skin cancer. I would encourage anyone who is interested in facial cancer and reconstruction to study carefully the works of these outstanding surgeons.

Foreword

It can be stated categorically that the concept and technique of flap transfer in the area of the face is superior to any other method of repair in respect to color-match, thickness, contour, stability, augmentation and conformation and cosmesis. The concept and the technique have therefore become axiomatic for the rehabilitation of surgical wounds in the area of the face. Recognition of the practicality of the clinical application of these flaps has enhanced the management of these cases to a significant degree.

This book is set within the framework of this recognition, giving a special emphasis to the rich variety of possibilities available to rehabilitate wounds in the area of the head and neck. The flaps that have been chosen and demonstrated are ones that have been developed over years of trial and error and proved to have the best chance of accomplishing a successful esthetic and functional repair. In this area of surgical activity, which is so uniquely topographical and endowed with such a rich blood supply, there are of course other varieties of flaps and other surgical techniques available. All of these possibilities enrich the craftsmanship and add a creative force to the process, and establish the "state of the art." The arrangement and qualities of this book assist in this endeavor.

Eleven chapters classify the surgical problems in specific anatomical regions with relevance to organ anatomy, spelling out graphically both the problem and its method of resolution. This is carried out within the framework of specific critical regions of the face, thus creating an optimal program for rehabilitation. The realistic use of immediate and regional tissues for repair almost always gives the best result. The photographic documentation of the great variety of surgical wounds about the face graphically supports this proposition.

The admonition in the last chapter on "Surgical Risks," that a recognition of possible risks, a means of keeping them at a minimum, and their resolution, gives balance to the book. The untrammelled directness of the arrangement of the book and its presentation helps the senior surgeons with a refreshment of their experience, and assists the younger surgeons with knowledgable support in the often puzzling problems of how to do the best repair with the most assurance on the level of high professionalism.

John Conley, M. D.

Preface

Local and regional skin flaps provide the basic foundation of facial reconstructive surgery. This fact has become axiomatic and is well recognized by studious practitioners of the craft. Skin flaps provide nondelayed, rapid reconstruction with abundant tissue, giving an excellent color match with the surrounding tissue and an adequate blood supply when performed properly and without complications. This monograph will begin with a chapter outlining a basic classification of facial flaps as to their blood supply, geometry and design, and site of origin. This will be followed by chapters describing the various facial flaps which have been found to be most useful by the author in facial reconstruction. No attempt has been made to present every flap that has been described in the world literature. Only flaps that have proven their usefulness and reliability will be described. The earlier chapters will deal with random flaps, deriving their blood supply from the sub-dermal plexus, and this will be followed by chapters on axial pattern and regional flaps. Following the chapters on individual flaps will be a chapter regarding major reconstructive efforts when more than one flap is required or when another method of reconstruction is combined with a skin flap. The last chapter, perhaps the most important in the book, will deal with the complications of facial flaps. This general subject has been largely ignored in the literature to this point in time, although occasional case reports of complications can be found. The emphasis in this chapter will be placed on the prevention of complications of facial flaps and the specific treatment of these untoward occurrences.

On the theory that one picture is worth a thousand words (to which the author generally subscribes), the publishers have kindly consented to supplement the text liberally with illustrations that will demonstrate the design and execution as well as the postoperative results of all the surgical procedures described. The chapter on complications will also be adequately illustrated.

This work deals only with flaps in facial reconstruction. It does not address many other useful reconstructive modalities such as skin grafts, composite grafts, homografts and alloplastic implants, all of which have their specific indications and applications. The reader should study and have a thorough understanding of the basic anatomy of the face and neck and the physiology of facial flaps which are covered in other authoritative works on this subject.

Most of the reconstructions discussed in this book were performed following the removal of skin cancer. A facial flap reconstruction should not be undertaken unless it is reasonably assured that tumor removal has been complete. The subject of tumor extirpation is not addressed in this work but should be thoroughly understood before these types of reconstructions are attempted following tumor removal.

All of the cases illustrated in this work are those of the author unless otherwise noted in the figure legends.

1 Classifications of Facial Flaps

For the purpose of this monograph, facial skin flaps will be classified according to their blood supply (random pattern versus axial pattern) and according to their method of design and execution. A final method of classification might involve the region of location of the donor tissues for the flaps. Most of the random pattern flaps are local flaps whereas the axial pattern flaps are regional or distant flaps.

CLASSIFICATION ACCORDING TO BLOOD SUPPLY[1]

Random Pattern Flaps

A random pattern flap receives its blood supply from segmental or axial arteries which lie deep to the muscular layer and send perpendicular perforating branches through the muscle and into the subcutaneous tissue at the base of the flap. These perforating vessels feed the dermal-subdermal plexus, which nourishes the skin of the flap. Most of the local facial flaps discussed in this volume are random pattern flaps (Figure 1).

Axial Pattern Flaps

An axial pattern flap receives its blood supply through a direct named cutaneous artery, which arises from an axial artery. This direct cutaneous artery lies above the muscle layer on the deep surface of the subcutaneous tissue. This artery connects directly to the dermal-subdermal plexus of the skin of the flap. Because of the direct axial blood flow pattern, this type of flap can survive up to a length of 50 percent greater than a random pattern flap of similar size.[1] Many of the regional flaps discussed in this volume will be axial pattern flaps (Figure 2).

CLASSIFICATION ACCORDING TO DESIGN AND EXECUTION

Rotation Flaps

A rotation flap is a semi-circular flap of skin and subcutaneous tissue that rotates about a pivot point into a defect to be closed. The donor site is usually closed by direct suture of the wound, or by a skin graft when direct closure is impossible (Figure 3).

Transposition Flaps

A transposition flap consists of a segment of skin and subcutaneous tissue that is elevated and then transposed over an intervening bridge of normal undisturbed skin into a defect. The donor defect is closed directly (Figure 4) or with a graft (Figure 5).

Interpolation Flaps

An interpolation flap consists of a segment of skin and subcutaneous tissue which is elevated and advanced or rotated into a nearby defect that is not immediately adjacent to the donor area. The pedicle of the flap passes over or under the intervening tissue (Figure 6).

Advancement Flaps

An advancement flap is composed of a segment of skin and subcutaneous tissue that is moved directly into a defect without any rotation, transposition or interpolation. Most of these are single pedicle advancement flaps (Figure 7) or V-to-Y advancement flaps. Occasionally a bipedicle advancement flap is utilized.

CLASSIFICATION ACCORDING TO TISSUES COMPOSING FACIAL FLAPS

Facial flaps composed of other tissues in addition to skin and subcutaneous tissue are classified as compound flaps. Compound flaps that have been found to be most useful in facial reconstruction are musculocutaneous (skin-muscle) flaps, and several of these will be described in subsequent chapters. Flaps containing cartilage or bone are other examples of compound flaps.

REFERENCE

1. Grabb WC, Myer MB: Skin Flaps. Boston: Little Brown & Co, 1975

2 Facial Reconstruction with Local and Regional Flaps

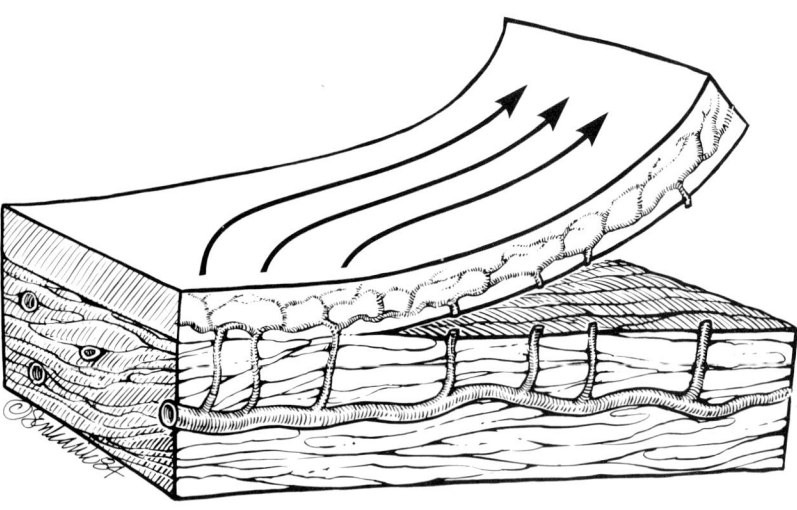

Figure 1. Random Pattern Flap.

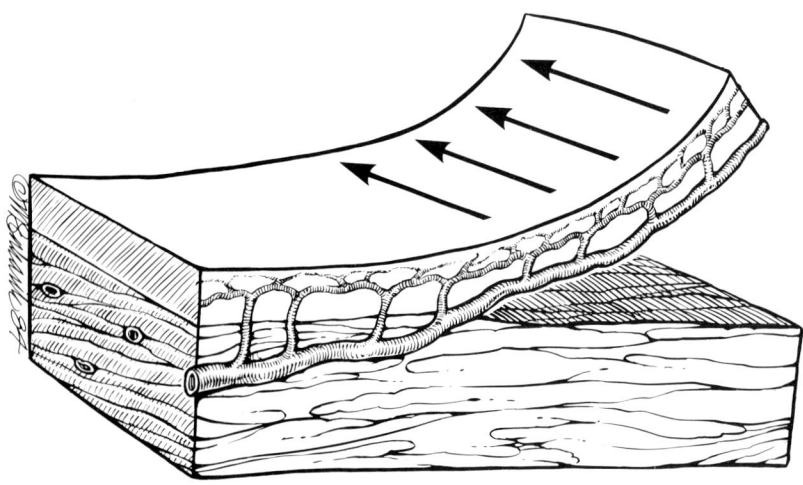

Figure 2. Axial Pattern Flap.

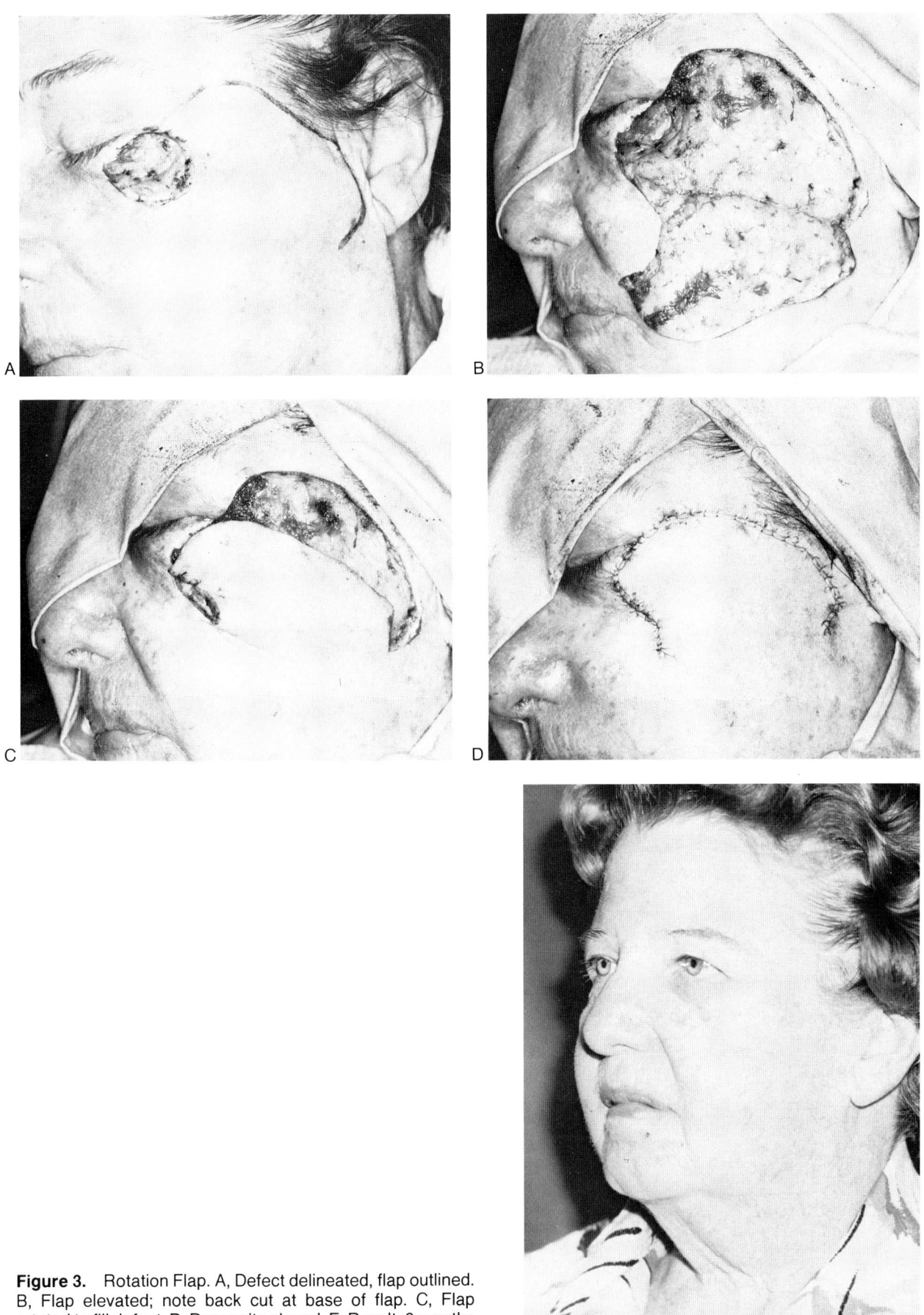

Figure 3. Rotation Flap. A, Defect delineated, flap outlined. B, Flap elevated; note back cut at base of flap. C, Flap rotated to fill defect. D, Donor site closed. E, Result, 6 months postoperative.

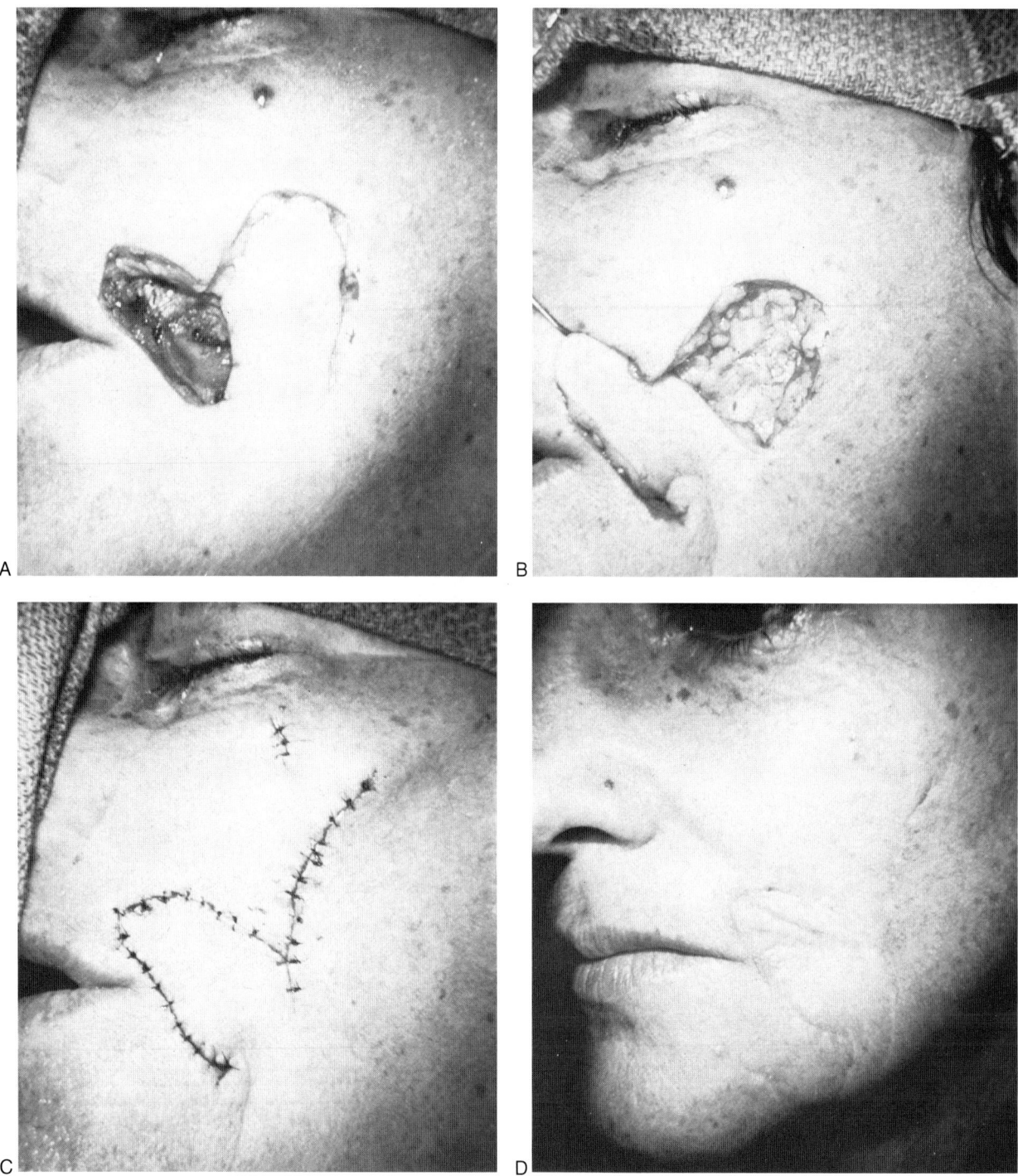

Figure 4. Transposition Flap. A, Defect delineated, transposition flap incised and elevated. B, Flap transposed into defect. C, Donor site and flap closed. D, Result, 6 months postoperative.

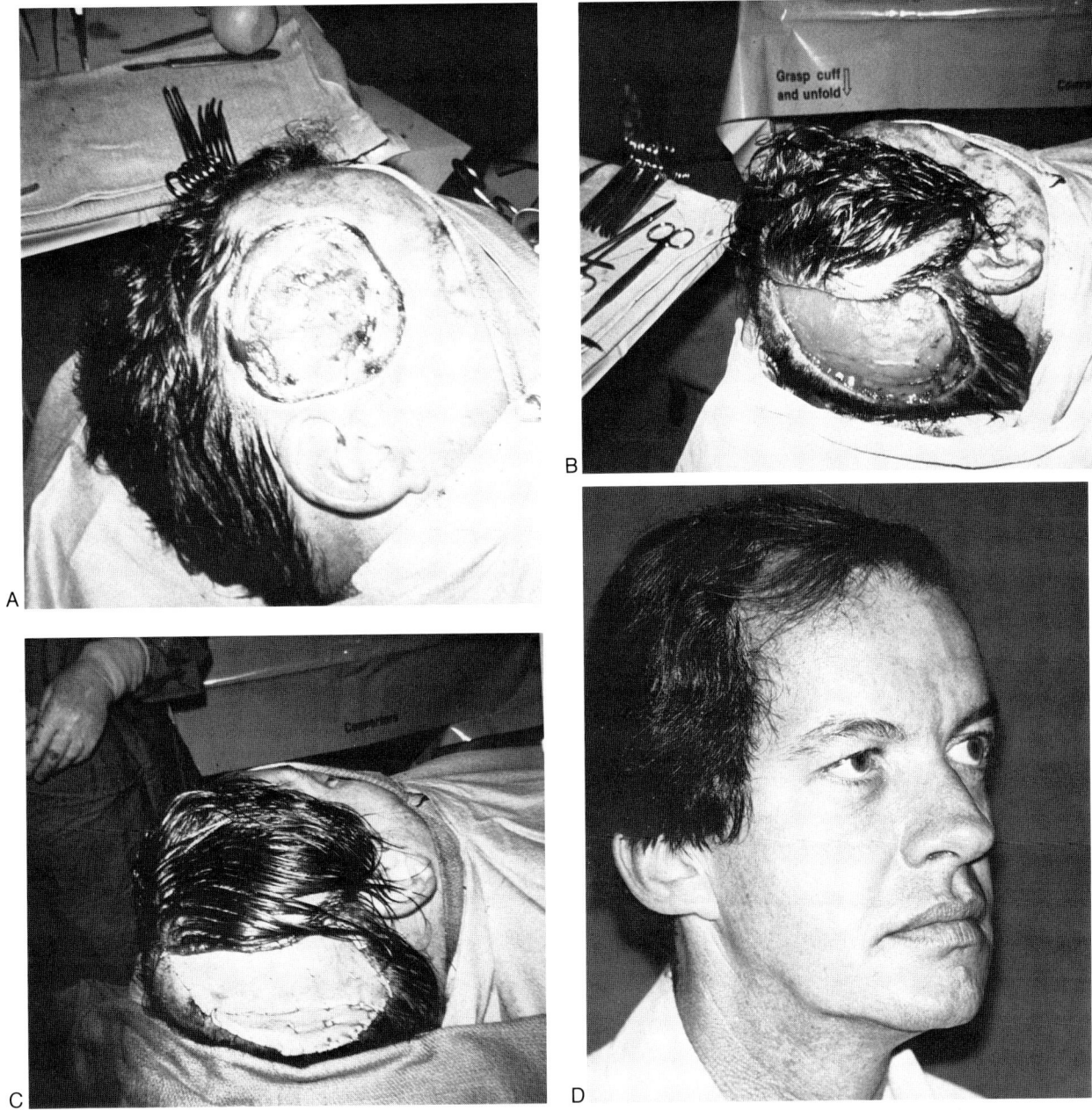

Figure 5. Transposition Flap. A, Large defect created by excision of invasive malignant melanoma. B, Large superiorly-based, hair-bearing scalp flap transposed over ear into defect. C, Donor site closed with split-thickness skin graft. D, Final result, 6 months postoperative.

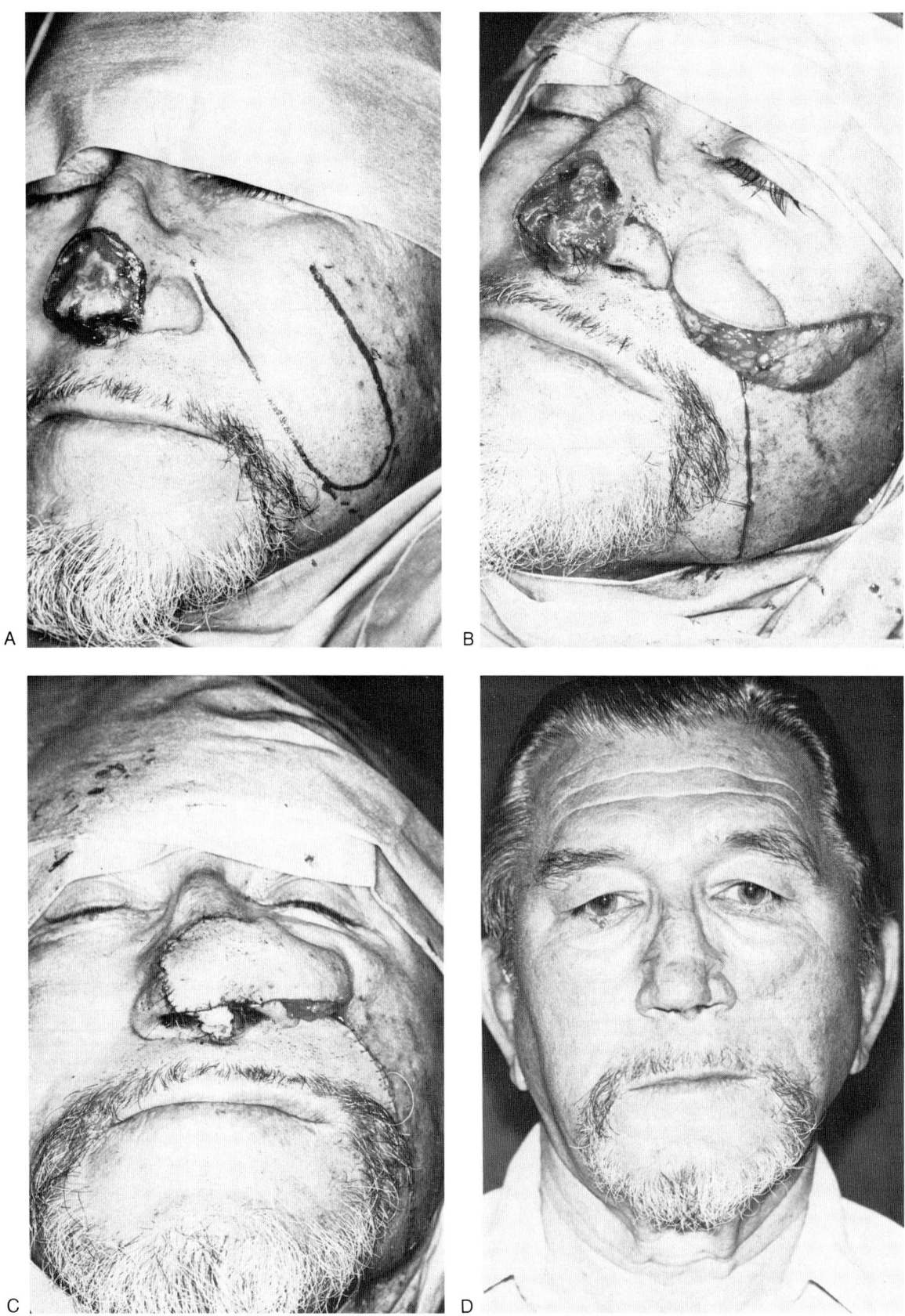

Figure 6. Interpolation Flap. A, Nasal tip defect created by Mohs' excision of recurrent basal carcinoma, nasolabial flap outlined. B, Flap raised, donor site closed directly. C, Nasolabial flap interpolated to nasal defect, base of flap divided and revised 2 weeks postoperatively. D, Final result, 6 months postoperative.

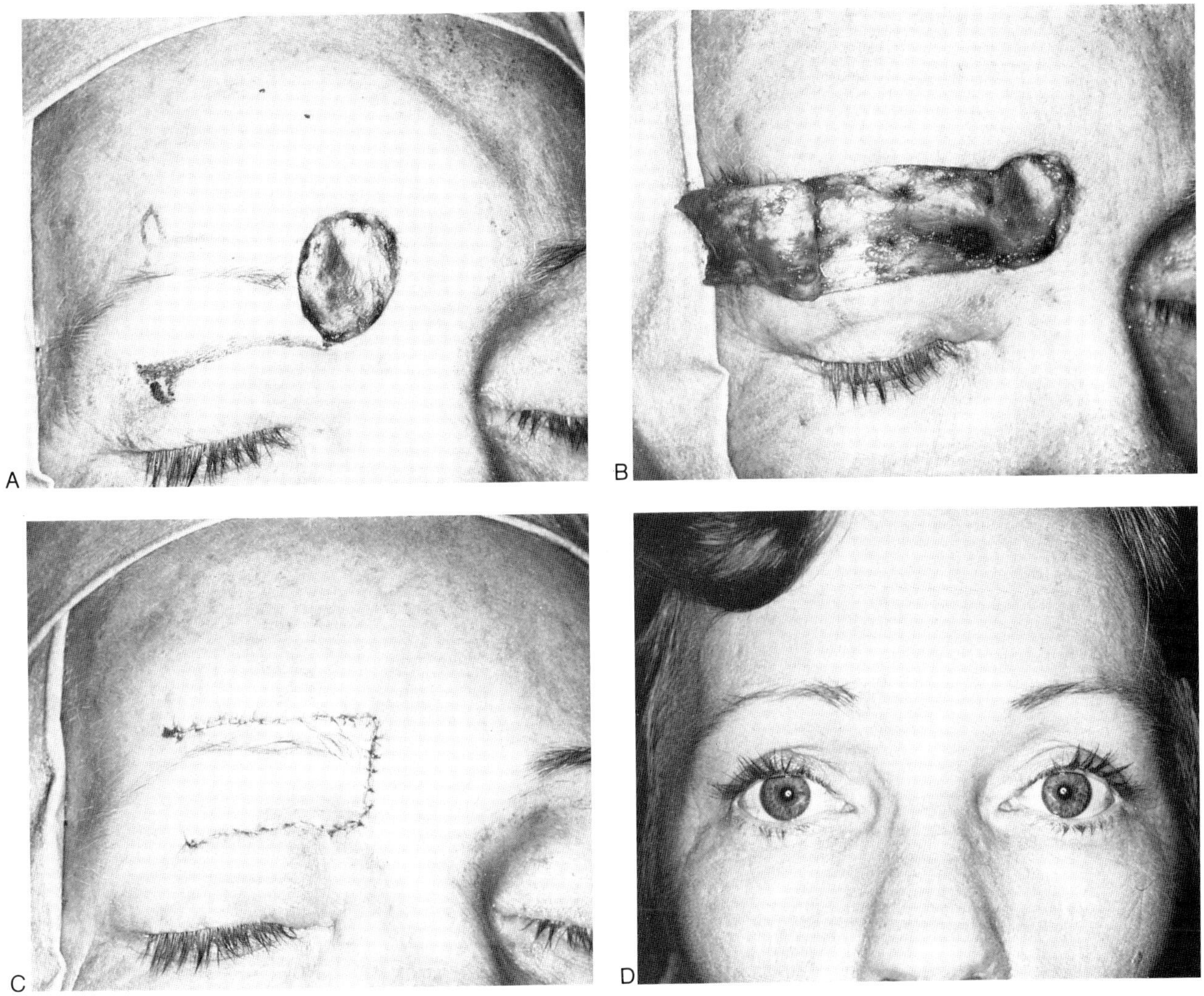

Figure 7. Advancement Flap. A, Defect created by excision of large primary basal cell carcinoma, advancement flap outlined. B, Flap elevated in subcutaneous plane superficial to orbicularis muscle and supraorbital neurovascular pedicle. C, Flap advanced to fill defect including advancement of medial brow. D, Result, 6 months postoperative.

2 Nasolabial Flaps

Medial cheek tissue located lateral to the nasolabial crease has been used for mid-facial reconstruction since the earliest descriptions of facial flaps.[1,2] Many nasolabial flaps have been devised and they are probably the most widely used and useful flaps for nasal reconstruction. The nasolabial crease is formed by the junction of the upper lip and lower nose with the cheek. It is created by the insertion of several of the mimetic facial muscles into the skin of the lip at this juncture. The forces of muscle contraction and gravity with time create a fold of skin lateral to this crease in the area of the medial cheek, which is called the nasolabial cheek fold. There is abundant, non-hairbearing skin in this area, particularly in older individuals. The cheek in this region has an extensive and excellent blood supply from branches of the facial artery and is drained by the facial and angular veins. Because of this rich blood supply, nasolabial flaps may be based superiorly or inferiorly and, if properly designed will rarely fail in a suitable host. Abundant tissue is usually available in the nasolabial area, and the size of the flap is limited only by the amount of cheek tissue which can be used in the flap and still affect a primary closure of the donor site in the nasolabial crease. Because the crease is a prominent facial landmark, the donor site closure is usually easily hidden in this area.

Nasolabial flaps are used most often for the reconstruction of defects created by the excision of facial skin malignancies. For this reason, determination of precise measurements of the flap cannot be taken until the dimensions of the recipient area have been assured. An appropriately wide excision is marked surrounding the lesion and a flap to fit this defect, or slightly larger, is usually marked. After the tumor margins have been cleared and the size of the defect determined, the flap is raised. Occasionally the area of the proposed flap will have to be revised when the defect is larger than anticipated (Figure 8). Generally, the flap should be kept thin and consist of only skin and subdermal fat. If a significant amount of nasal cartilage or bone has been removed, the flap can be made thicker to fill in this deformity.

SUPERIORLY-BASED NASOLABIAL FLAPS

The superiorly-based nasolabial flap is most useful for central and lateral nasal dorsal defects and defects of the nasal alae and tip. The only area of the nose where this flap is not useful is the more superior area. Carrying the flap too far superiorly can give rise to a medial lower eyelid ectropion when the donor site is closed.

After the flap has been designed and the defect size determined, the flap is raised in the mid-subcutaneous plane, carefully preserving the subdermal plexus. Dissection is continued in the same plane out into the lateral cheek (Figure 9B) as far as is necessary to move the flap medially to the defect and close the donor site. The lateral limb of the flap is kept as short as possible and can always be lengthened as the procedure goes on. Making the lateral limb too long will narrow the base and could compromise the blood supply of the flap. After the flap has been transferred into the recipient area, the donor site is closed.

It is often necessary to remove a standing cutaneous cone (dog-ear) at the inferior limit of the donor site (Figure 9E,F). If this area has been incised in a pointed fashion, as in a fusiform excision, this step will often be unnecessary (Figure 10). Occasionally there is a standing cutaneous cone at the rotation point. The excision of this redundant tissue should always be carried out away from the base of the flap in order not to narrow the base, which carries the vascular supply of the flap (Figure 9C,D). If the defect on the nose directly abuts the flap, the procedure can be done in a single stage (Figures 8,9). If the flap does not immediately abut the defect and a narrow skin bridge separates the two, the bridge of skin can be excised for a one stage procedure (Figure 11). If the skin bridge is large and it is impractical to excise it, an interpolation flap is necessary, and a second stage to release the flap is required 10 to 21 days following the primary procedure (Figure 6). It should be noted that undermining done to close the flap donor defect is always carried out in a lateral direction. The skin medial to the nasolabial crease is not undermined in order not to distort the ala, lip or commissure. It should also be noted that the lateral ala is a fixed landmark, and as the defect becomes more inferior in location, a superiorly-based flap will have to twist around this fixed landmark and can cause distortion (Figure 12).

INFERIORLY-BASED NASOLABIAL FLAPS

The inferiorly-based nasolabial flap is most useful for defects of the upper lip, floor of the nose and columella. This flap is ideal for lateral upper lip defects involving only skin and muscle and not involving the vermilion of the lip (Figure 13).

The inferiorly-based flap is designed by marking out the proposed defect as before. The flap is marked along the nasolabial crease and up the lateral nasal crease in a pointed fashion (Figure 13A). The width of the flap is determined by the proposed height of the defect. It is imperative that the flap be as wide as the height of the lip defect or wider to insure that the verticle height of the lip is not shortened. After the size of the defect has been determined, the flap is elevated as before and rotated into place. The donor site is closed in the natural nasolabial crease and lateral nasal fold. The rotation point of the inferiorly-based flap is located around the angle of the mouth. Since this area is not a fixed point, it is usually capable of being repositioned without distorting the symmetry of the mouth. If this area is distorted, a secondary procedure can be carried out several weeks later to improve the appearance. If a skin bridge separates the defect from the inferiorly-based flap, the skin can be excised in the same way as for the superiorly-based flap (Figure 14).

Walkinshaw and Chaffee[3] recently addressed the problem of trap door contracture of nasolabial flaps encountered in their experience. This problem tended to occur in older men with thick nasal skin with considerable sebaceous hypertrophy. While the author has seen this problem (Figure 15), it does not seem to be as common as in their experience. Their solution was to excise the skin of the flap after it had healed and place a skin graft on the resulting defect. The author still prefers debulking procedures and revision of the unequal scars at the edges of the flap when these occur because the color and texture match of the flap itself is far superior to that of a skin graft in most cases.

REFERENCES

1. Cameron RR, Lathamid WD, Dowling, JA: Reconstruction of the nose and upper lip with nasolabial flaps. Plast Reconstr Surg 52:145, 1973
2. Pers M: Cheek flaps in partial rhinoplasty. Scand J Plast Reconstr Surg 1:37, 1967
3. Walkinshaw MD, Chaffee HH: The nasolabial flap: a problem and its correction. Plast Reconstr Surg 69:30–34, 1982

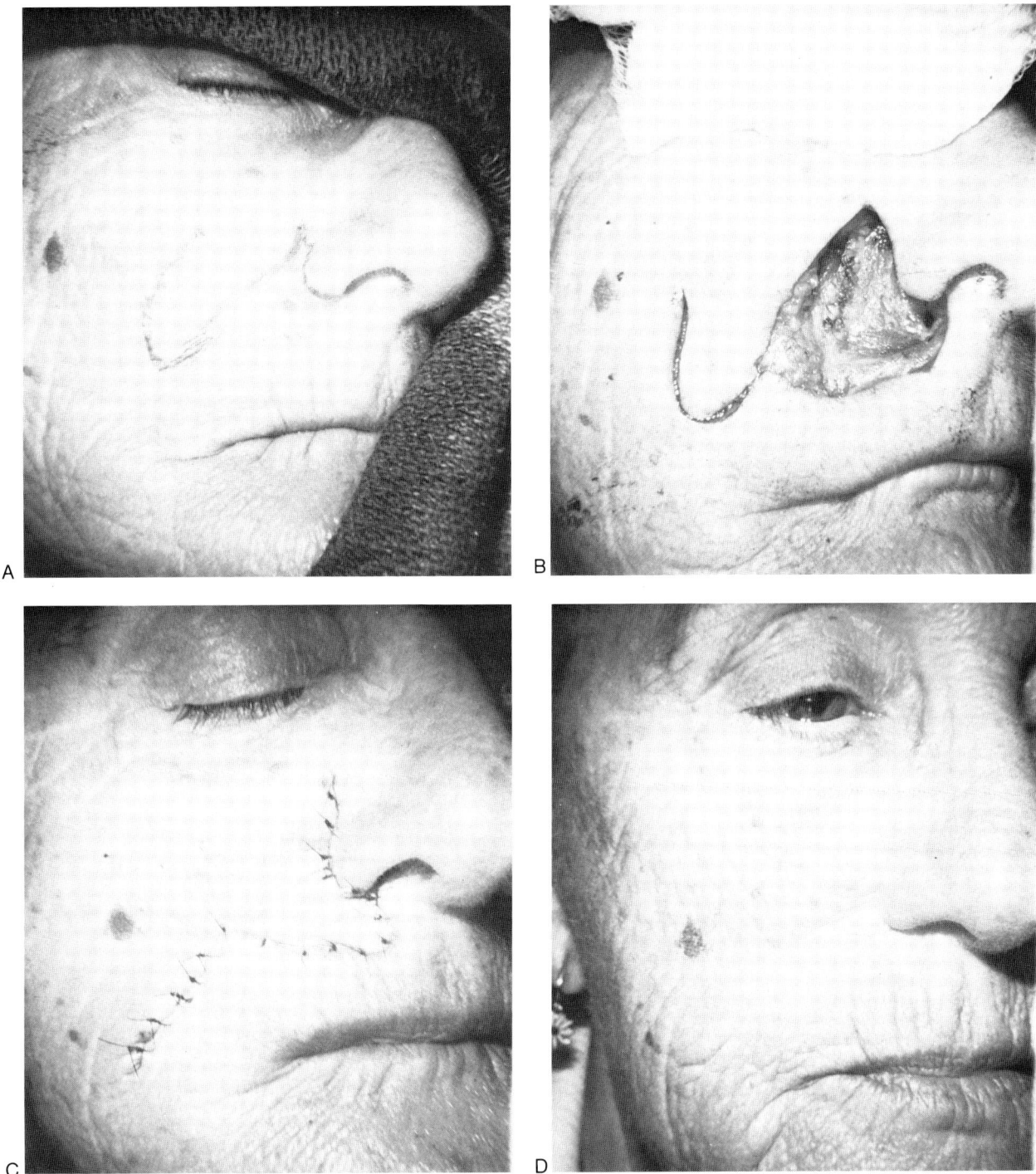

Figure 8. A, Proposed excision of recurrent basal cell carcinoma outlined, nasolabial flap marked. B, Tumor excision by microscopically controlled margins yielding a larger than anticipated defect. Note: nasolabial flap incised wider than previously anticipated. C, Flap rotated into place, donor site closed. D, Result, 3 years postoperative. (Reprinted with permission from: Becker FF: Local tissue flaps in reconstructive facial plastic surgery. South Med J 70:677–680, 1977)

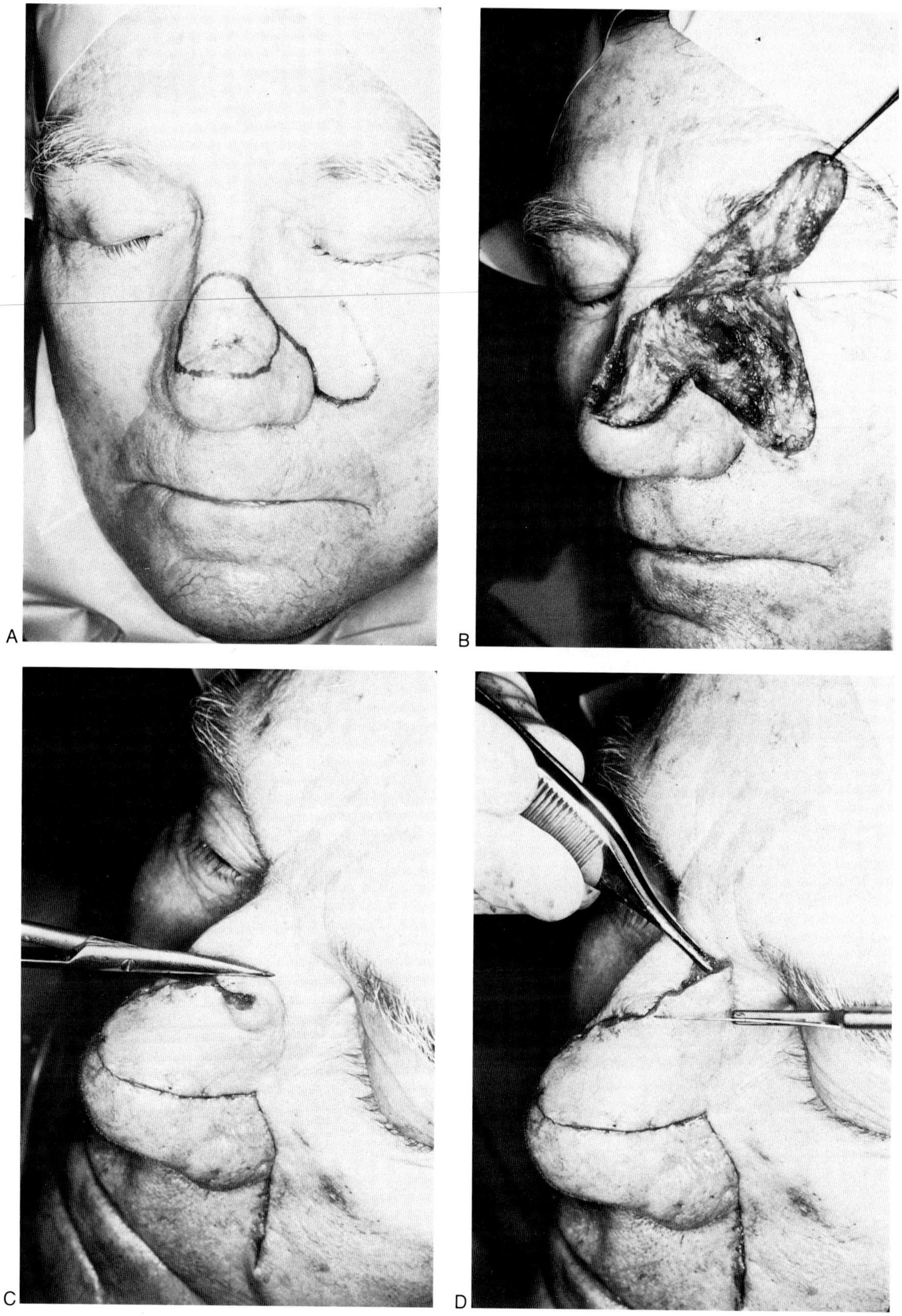

Figure 9. A, Proposed excision for recurrent basal cell carcinoma outlined, superiorly-based nasolabial flap marked. B, Flap raised, cheek undermined in subcutaneous plane. C, Standing cutaneous cone at rotation point of flap incised away from base of flap. D, Excision of redundant tissue.

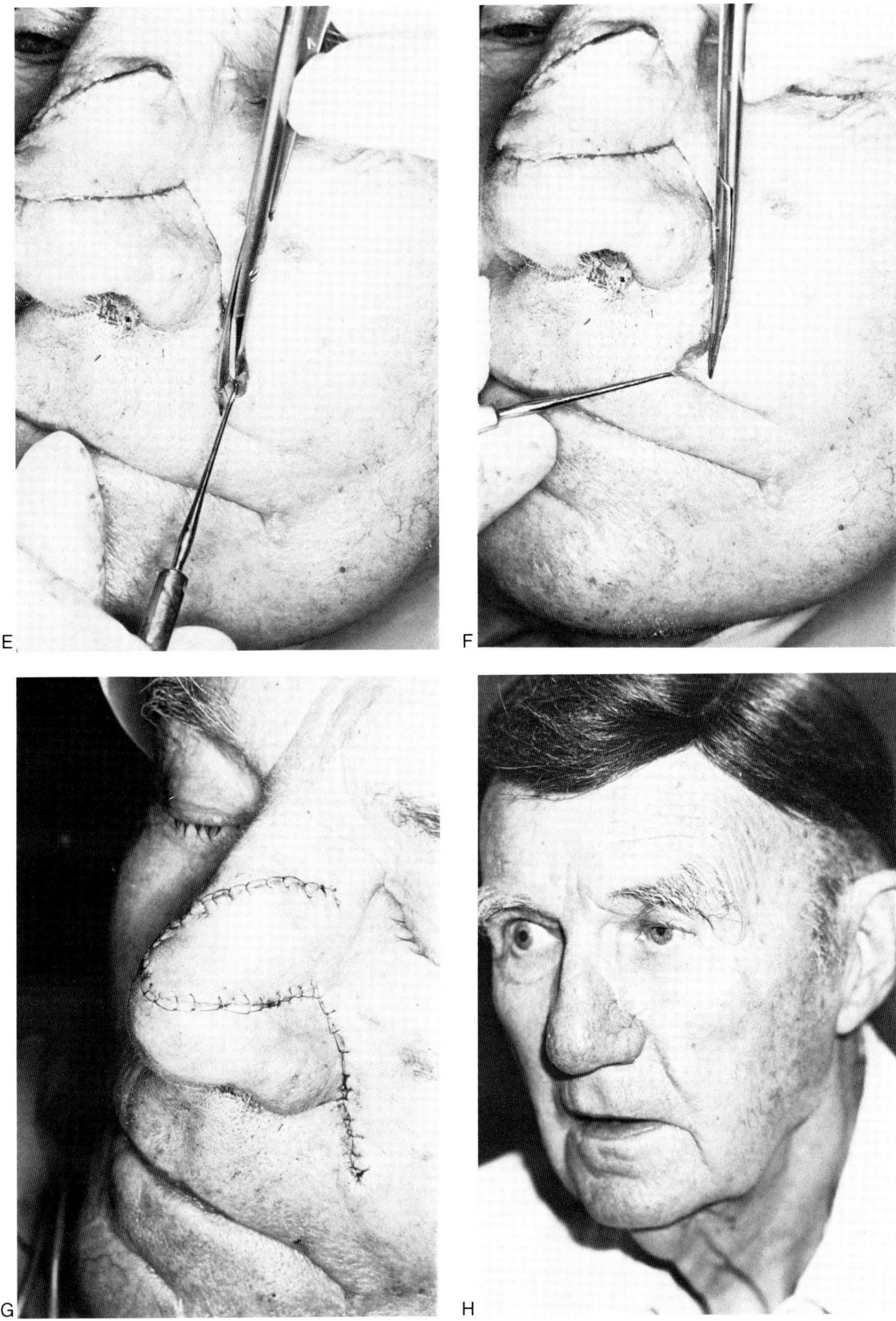

Figure 9. (cont.) E, Small standing cutaneous cone at distal end of donor site incised. F, Redundant tissue excised. G, Final closure. H, Results, 6 months postoperative.

14 Facial Reconstruction with Local and Regional Flaps

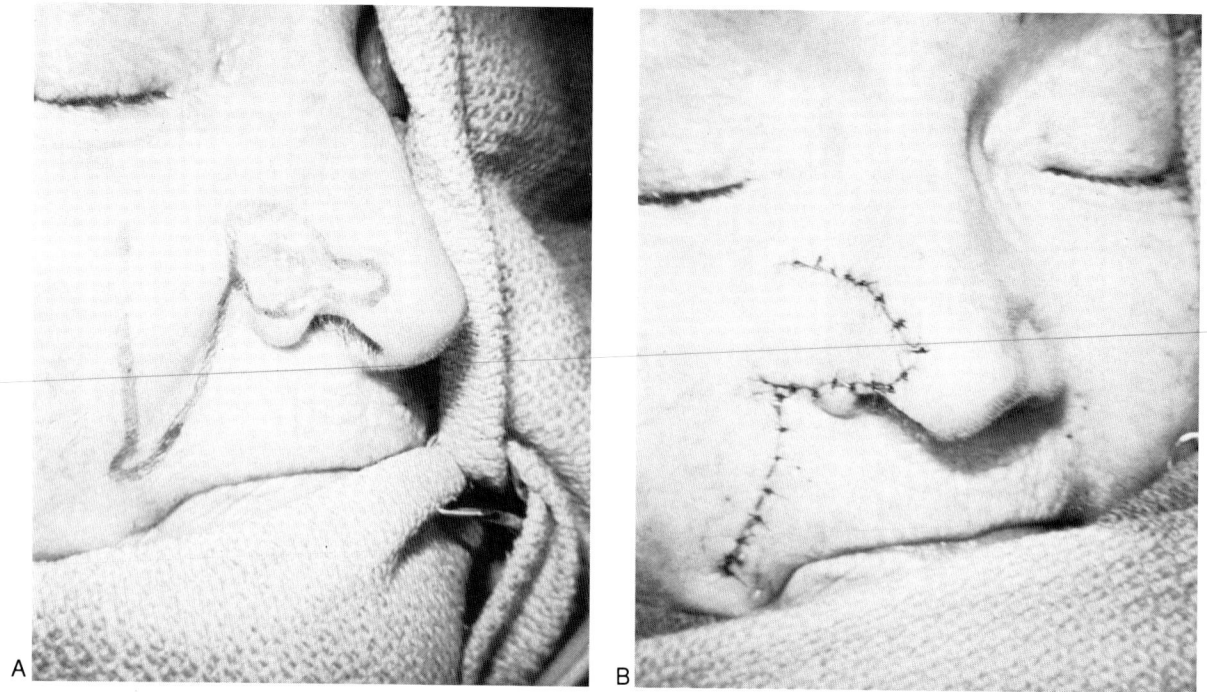

Figure 10. A, Donor site marked with a pointed end. B, This method obviates the removal of a standing cutaneous cone.

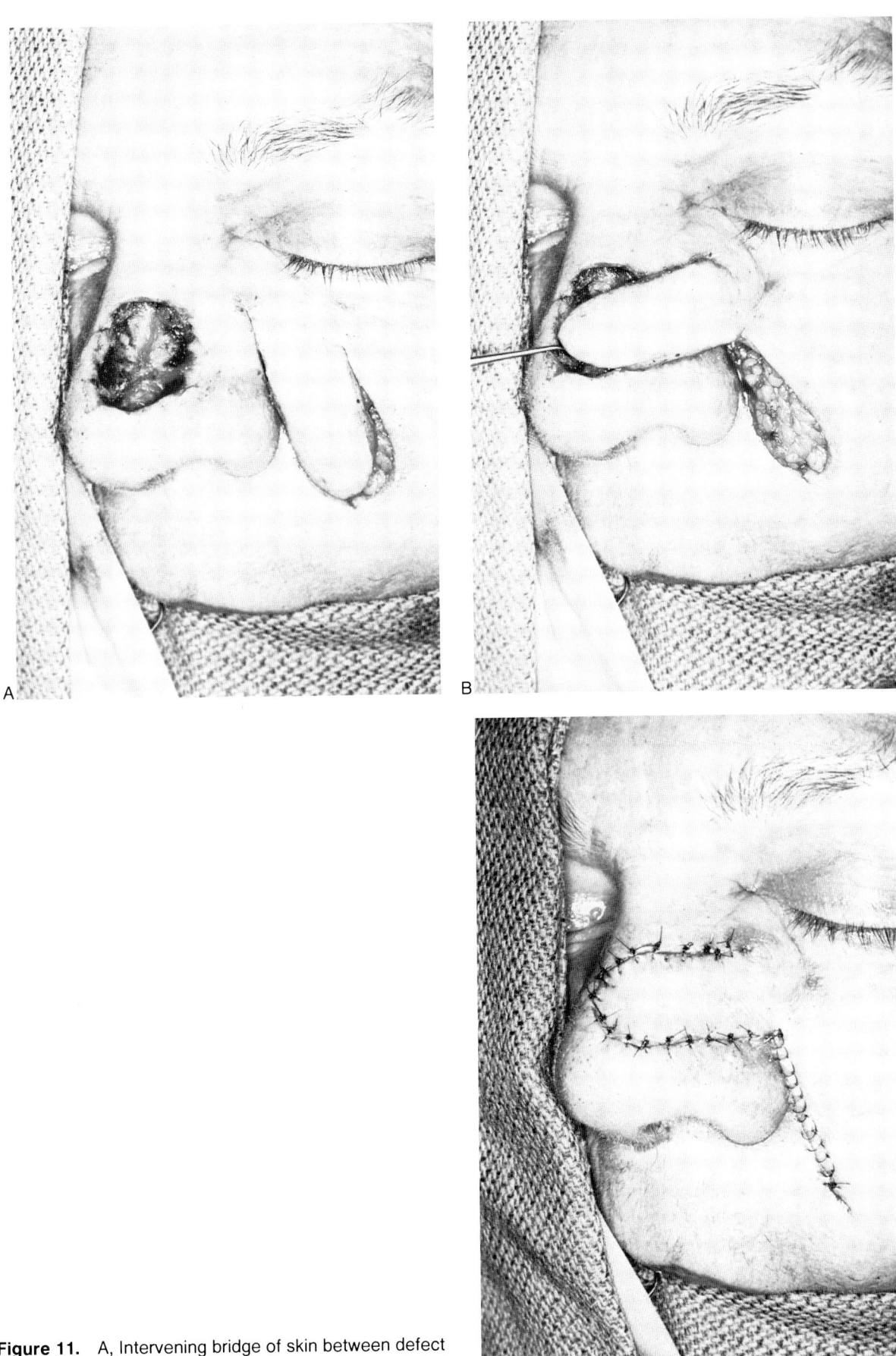

Figure 11. A, Intervening bridge of skin between defect and nasolabial flap. B, Skin bridge removed, flap rotated into place. C, Final closure.

16 Facial Reconstruction with Local and Regional Flaps

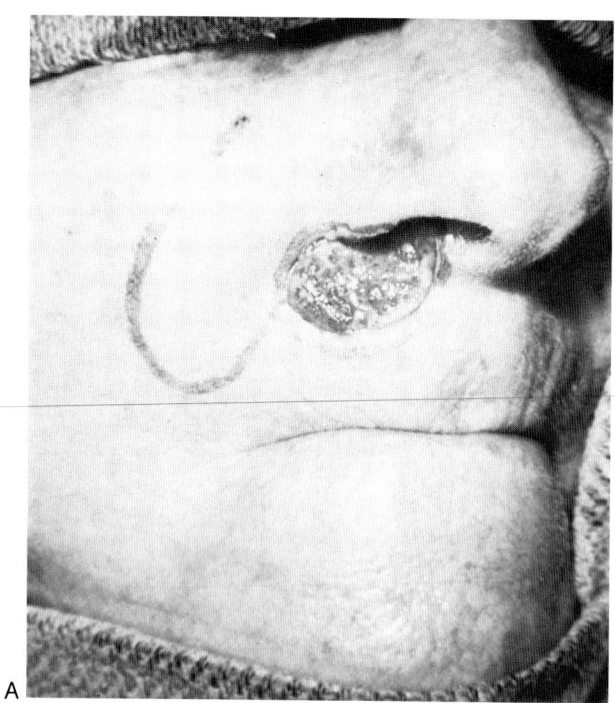

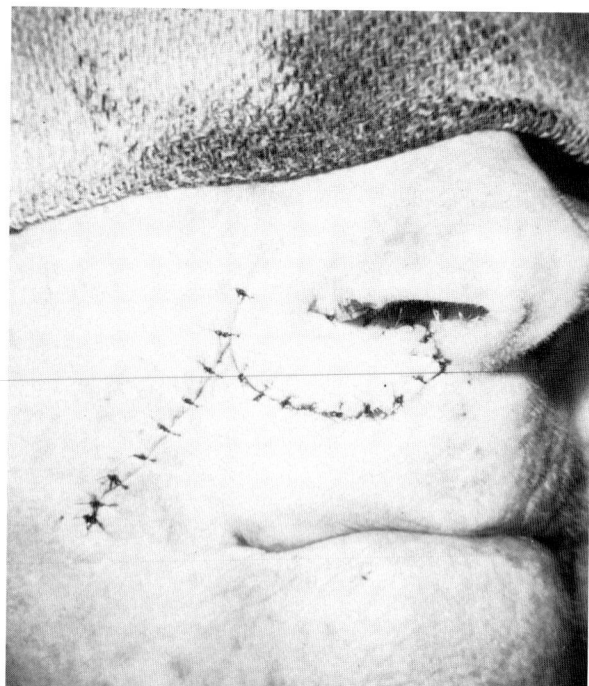

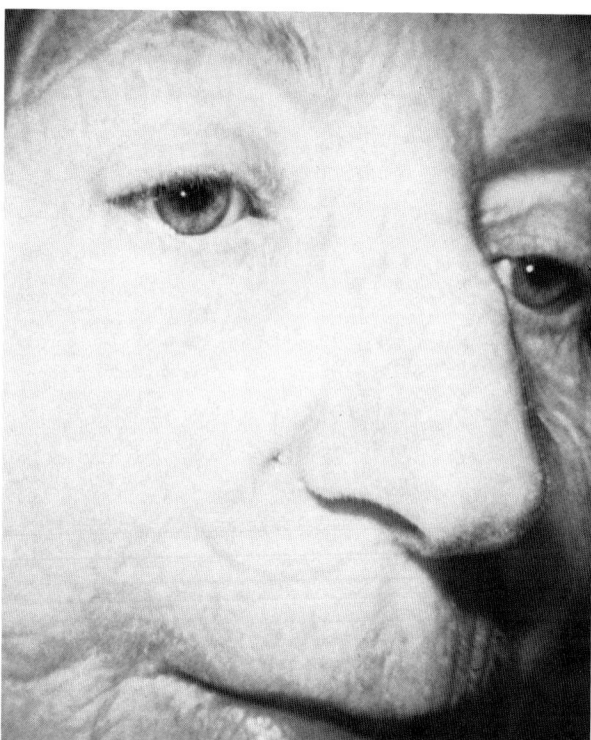

Figure 12. A, Superiorly-based nasolabial flap with base of flap in an inferior location for upper lip reconstruction. B, Flap twists around the ala, a fixed facial landmark. C, Slight distortion of flap 6 months postoperative. An inferiorly based flap might be more appropriate for this type of defect.

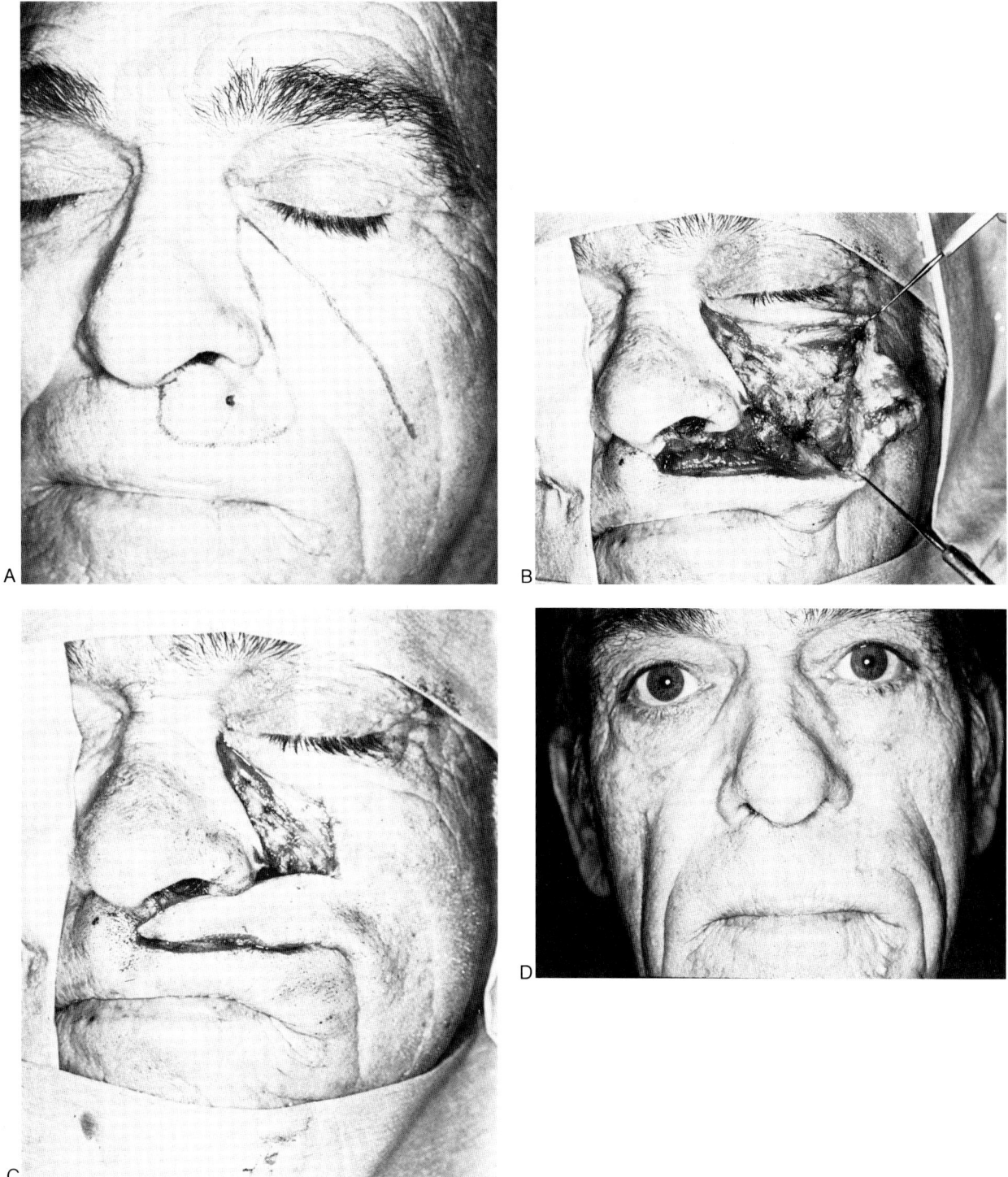

Figure 13. A, Proposed excision of tumor outlined, inferiorly-based nasolabial flap marked. B, Tumor excised, flap and lateral cheek undermined. C, Flap rotated into place, donor site close primarily. D, Result, 6 months postoperative.

18 Facial Reconstruction with Local and Regional Flaps

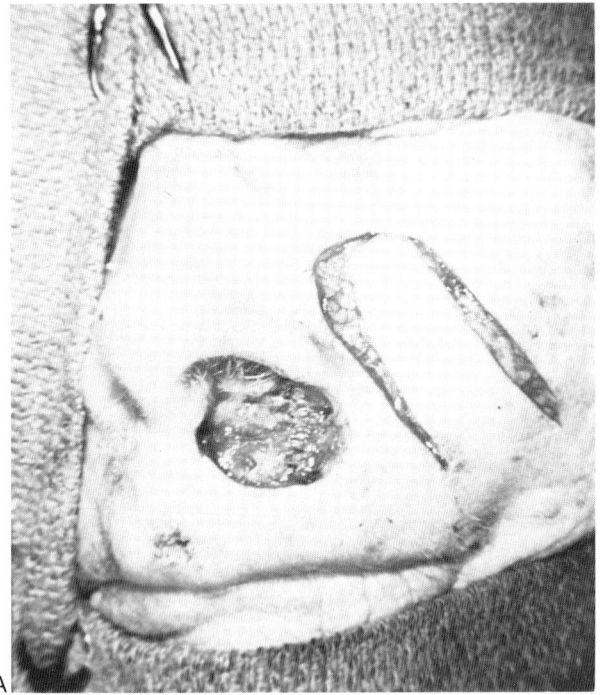
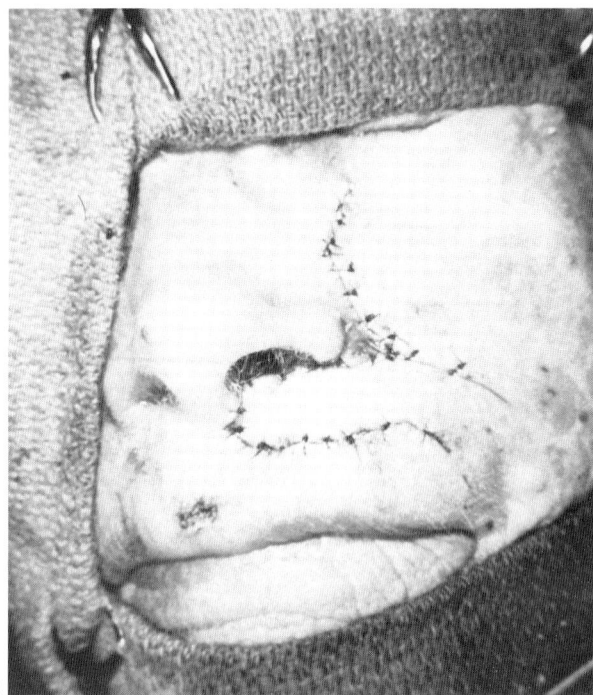
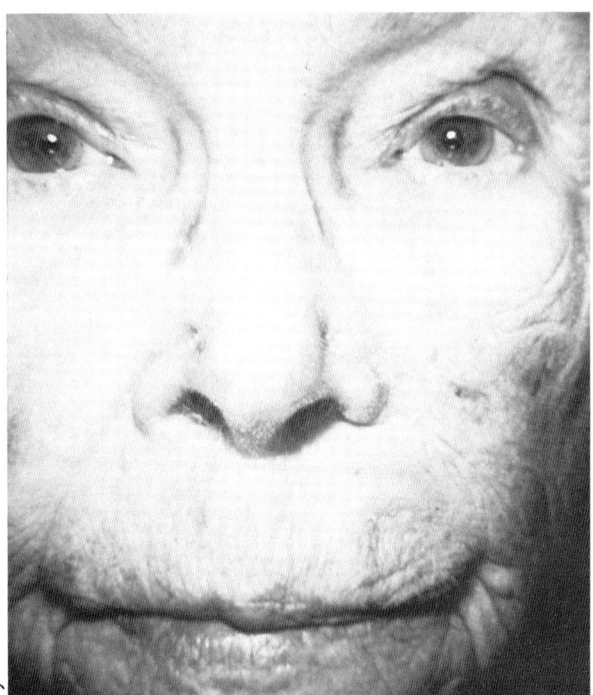

Figure 14. A, Defect separated from inferiorly-based nasolabial flap by a skin bridge. B, Bridge excised, flap rotated into place, donor site closed primarily. C, Result, 6 months postoperative.

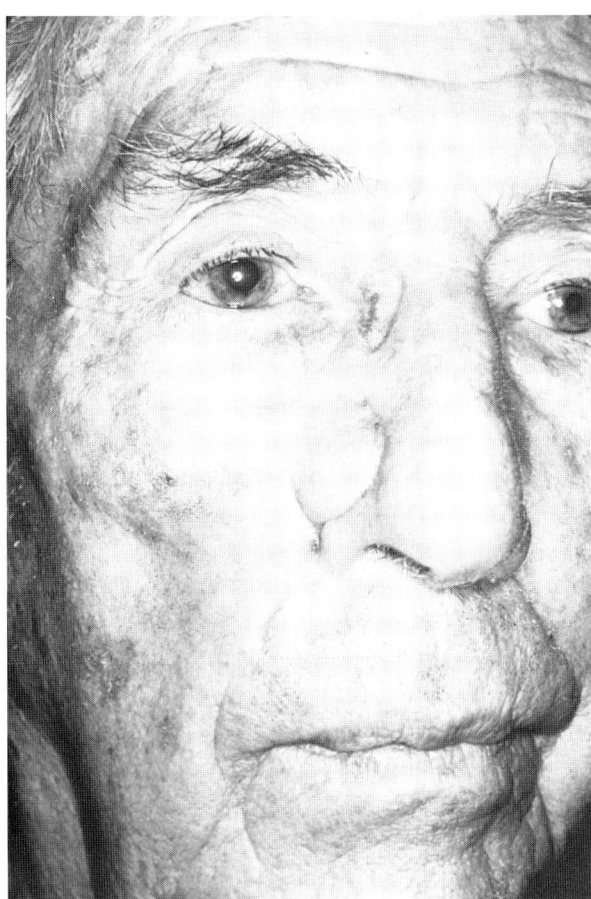
Figure 15. Inferiorly based nasolabial flap with trap door deformity in older male.

3 Cheek Flaps and Cervicofacial Flaps

The cheek and upper neck have the potential to provide an abundance of tissue to reconstruct moderate to large defects of the lateral nose, lateral upper lip and cheek. A variety of flap designs have been found to be useful and will be described. In addition to the excellent color match of this local tissue and the abundant blood supply secondary to broadly based flaps, other distinct advantages are provided by these flaps. They can be based inferiorly and anteriorly or superiorly and posteriorly. The scars created by the lines of closure tend to follow natural junctures of the face, such as the nasoalar groove, the nasolabial crease, the preauricular crease, and the infraorbital creases. This situation contrasts to some of the local facial flaps discussed elsewhere in this monograph, which by necessity often leave some scars running perpendicular to the lines of relaxed skin tension (*see* Chapter 5, Rhombic Flaps). When treating tumors that have a potential for metastasis, these flaps offer excellent exposure for the concomitant dissection of the parotid and cervical lymph node chains.[1]

ADVANCEMENT CHEEK FLAPS

The advancement cheek flap is most useful for a lateral nasal defect or a defect involving the lateral nose and adjacent cheek (Figure 16). The superior limb of the flap is placed in the natural infraorbital fold and is carried to a more superior location at the level of the lateral canthus to avoid an ectropion. The inferior limb is usually placed in the nasolabial crease. After the tumor has been excised and the area of the defect determined, the skin of the cheek is elevated in the subcutaneous plane as far laterally as is necessary to advance the flap to fill the nasal and/or cheek defect. A surprisingly abundant amount of tissue can be brought medially to fill in quite large defects, particularly in older individuals. Some redundancy at the lateral ends of the limbs of the flap can be dealt with as with any standing cutaneous cone. Occasionally, the dermis of the flap is tacked to the periosteum at the lateral nasal crease to make a natural fold in that area.

ROTATION CHEEK FLAPS

Tissues of the cheek may be rotated to fill in cheek, lip and nasal defects. These flaps are used much more frequently than advancement cheek flaps. Most frequently cheek flaps have an inferior base and are rotated forward to cover a more anteriorly located defect (Figure 17). Less often, the flap is based superiorly and is used to cover a defect of the medial cheek or chin.[2]

Inferiorly-Based Cheek Flaps

The inferiorly-based rotation cheek flap is useful for a defect of the medial cheek in the region of the nasolabial fold and is particularly suitable if the longest axis of the defect runs parallel to the fold. It is helpful to triangulate the proposed defect in such a way that its apex points downward and its base is in a superior location (Figure 17A). In planning the flap, it must be ascertained that the cheek tissue will be sufficiently mobile to rotate into the defect after wide undermining of the cheek skin. The outline of the flap curves backward and slightly upward from the defect to be closed. This line of the flap may be planned for an inferior defect as in Figure 17, or it may be in a more superior location in the infraorbital area for a more superior defect (Figure 18). If the superior edge of the flap is located in the area of the infraorbital rim, the extension of the flap posteriorly must be carried to the level of the lateral canthus and then back and anterior to the ear, if necessary. It is imperative to secure the dermis of the flap to the periosteum of the lateral orbital rim at the area of the lateral canthus to take tension off of the lower eyelid and prevent ectropion formation. McGregor[2] has correctly pointed out that the flap should be designed to rotate about a pivot point which lies along its baseline approximately midway between the extremes of the flap. The flap must be designed so that the distance between the pivot point and any point on the circumference of the flap before rotation equals the estimated distance after rotation. If the flap is not designed this way it could lead to unacceptable tension when the flap is transferred.

Once the defect is determined and the flap has been designed, the flap is raised in the subcutaneous plane superficial to the facial muscles. It is then rotated in to fill the defect and the edges of the flap are trimmed accordingly. After the flap has been rotated to fill the defect, a discrepancy is created in the lengths between the two sides of the line to be sutured at the donor site. The outer side is longer than the inner side. This discrepancy can be partially reduced by suturing under different tension on the two sides. If it is not possible to correct the discrepancy completely in that way, there are two other ways of correcting it. The first method of correcting this problem is with a back cut on the base of the flap (Figure 18D). This allows more equalization of the closure (Figure 18E). It must be remembered that this maneuver necessarily reduces the size of the base of the flap and thus its blood supply. However, these flaps ordinarily have sufficiently wide bases so that this is not a significant problem. The second method of dealing with the unequal lengths of the sides of the closure is by excising a triangle of skin along the outer side of the donor site. The most inconspicuous area to excise this triangle of skin and leave an unnoticeable scar is in the infraauricular area (Figure 19A). This is probably the best of these alternative methods in that the base of the flap is not compromised and the resulting scar is more easily camouflaged.

This is a flap that works well in most cases. McGregor found that the inferiorly-based rotation cheek flap had a higher record of necrosis than most any other facial flap.[2] This has not been the author's experience. The cheek rotation flap has had an excellent record with a high degree of reliability.

CERVICOFACIAL FLAPS

When larger defects are encountered in the medial cheek and lateral nasal and lip areas, the aforementioned cheek flaps can be carried into the neck for the movement of greater amounts of tissue. When this is the case, these flaps become cervicofacial flaps. The most commonly used cervicofacial flaps are based anteriorly and inferiorly (Figure 19), and less commonly they are based posteriorly and superiorly (Figure 20).

Anteriorly-Based Cervicofacial Flaps

The anteriorly-based cervicofacial flap is an excellent technique for the correction of larger defects of the nasoalar groove and medial cheek. It is basically an extension of the inferiorly-based cheek flap into the neck to obtain additional cervical skin to increase the size of the defect that can be closed. This flap takes advantage of the abundant tissues of the mandibulomasseteric jowl, which is particularly plentiful in older patients. The flap can also be extended to correct defects of the upper lip in addition to defects of the nasoalar groove and medial cheek, as is the case in Figure 21. The rotation point of the flap is often at the angle of the mouth, and occasionally a revisional operation will be necessary in this area (Figure 21G–I).

The anteriorly-based cervicofacial flap can be designed in such a way as to utilize the bilobed concept, which is discussed in some detail in Chapter 6. The design is illustrated in Figure 22, where a second lobe of the flap from the postauricular area is used to reconstruct partially the anterior cheek defect.

Weisberger and Hanke[1] have pointed out that there are some problems encountered in the use of this reconstructive technique. Even with very careful planning and execution, the forces of scar tissue contraction can cause deviations of important landmarks, particularly ectropion of the lower eyelid. This possibility should not preclude the use of this flap, but rather one should be prepared to deal with the eventuality of such a complication if it occurs (Figure 22E–J).

Posteriorly-Based Cervicofacial Flaps

The cervicofacial flap based posteriorly is used much less commonly than that which is based anteriorly and inferiorly. However, there are times in which this flap is particularly useful and Figure 20 is an excellent example of this. In this particular case, most of the tissue of the cheek was removed in treating a deeply invasive malignant melanoma. The raising of this flap provided a wide exposure of the parotid gland and upper neck for parotidectomy in conjunction with the reconstructive procedure. Excision of the tumor required removal of the lobule and inferior portion of the external ear. The standing cutaneous cone at the pivot point just under the ear provided an excellent method for reconstructing the lower ear and lobule (Figure 20D, E).

REFERENCES

1. Weisberger EL, Hanke W: Reconstruction of full-thickness defects of the cheek. Arch Otolaryngol 109:190–194, 1983
2. McGregor IA: Local skin flaps in facial reconstruction. Otolaryngol Clin North Am 15:77–98, 1982

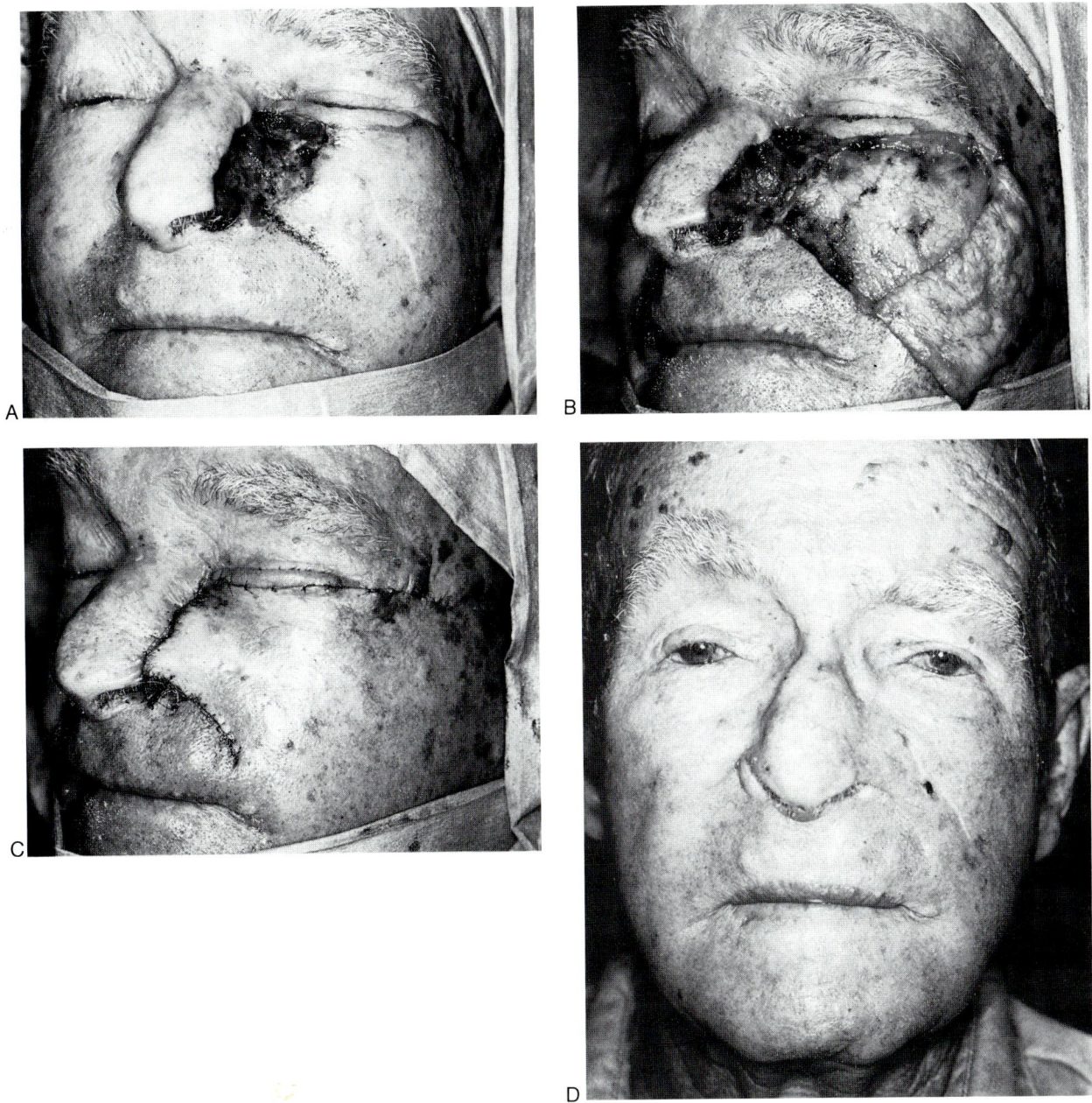

Figure 16. A, Defect of lateral nose and adjacent cheek, advancement cheek flap outlined. B, Flap elevated in subcutaneous plane onto lateral cheek. C, Flap advanced to fill defect. D, Final result, 8 months postoperative.

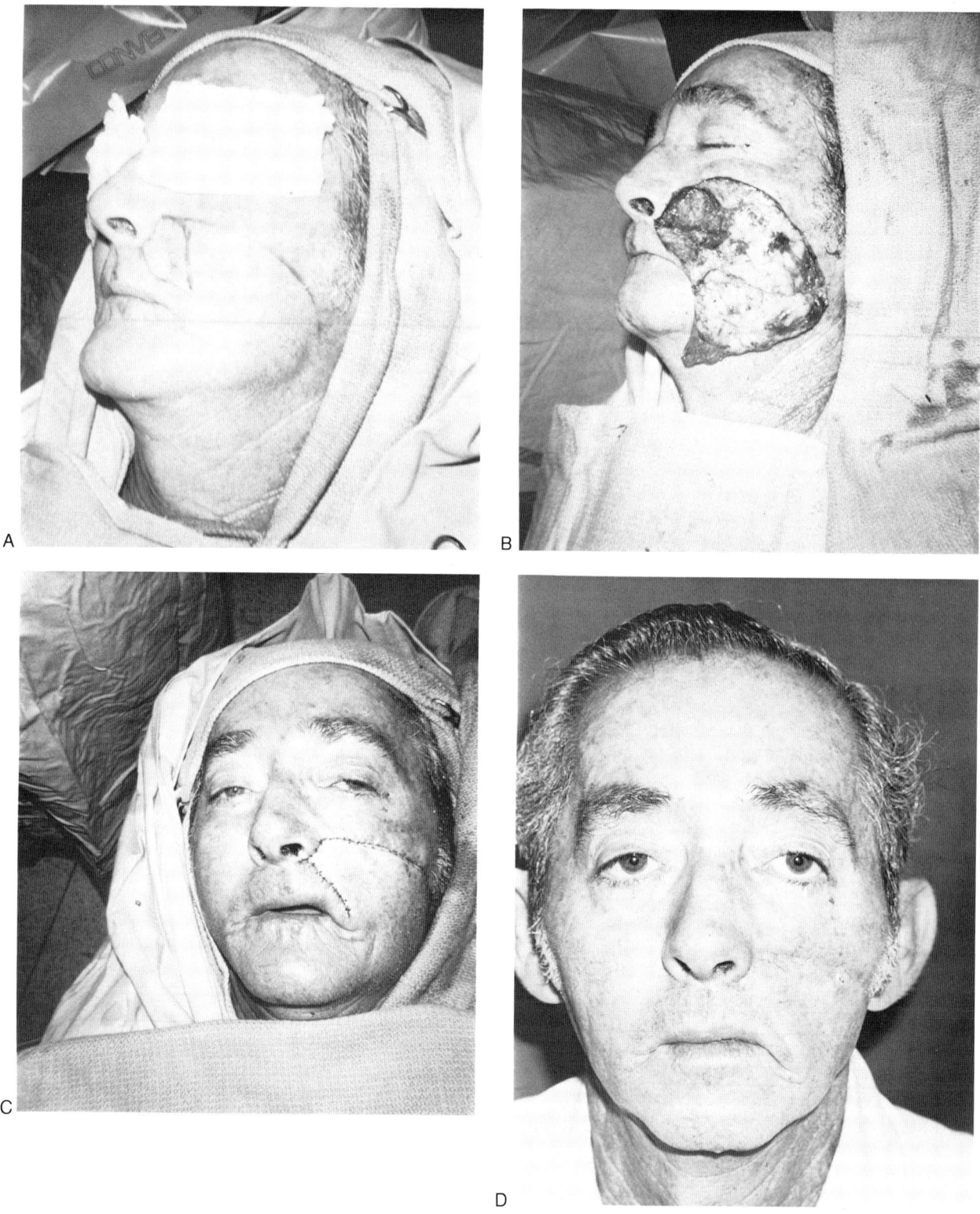

Figure 17. A, Proposed defect outlined with base superiorly and apex pointing inferiorly. B, Incisions made, flap elevated. C, Flap rotated into place. D, Final result, 6 months postoperative.

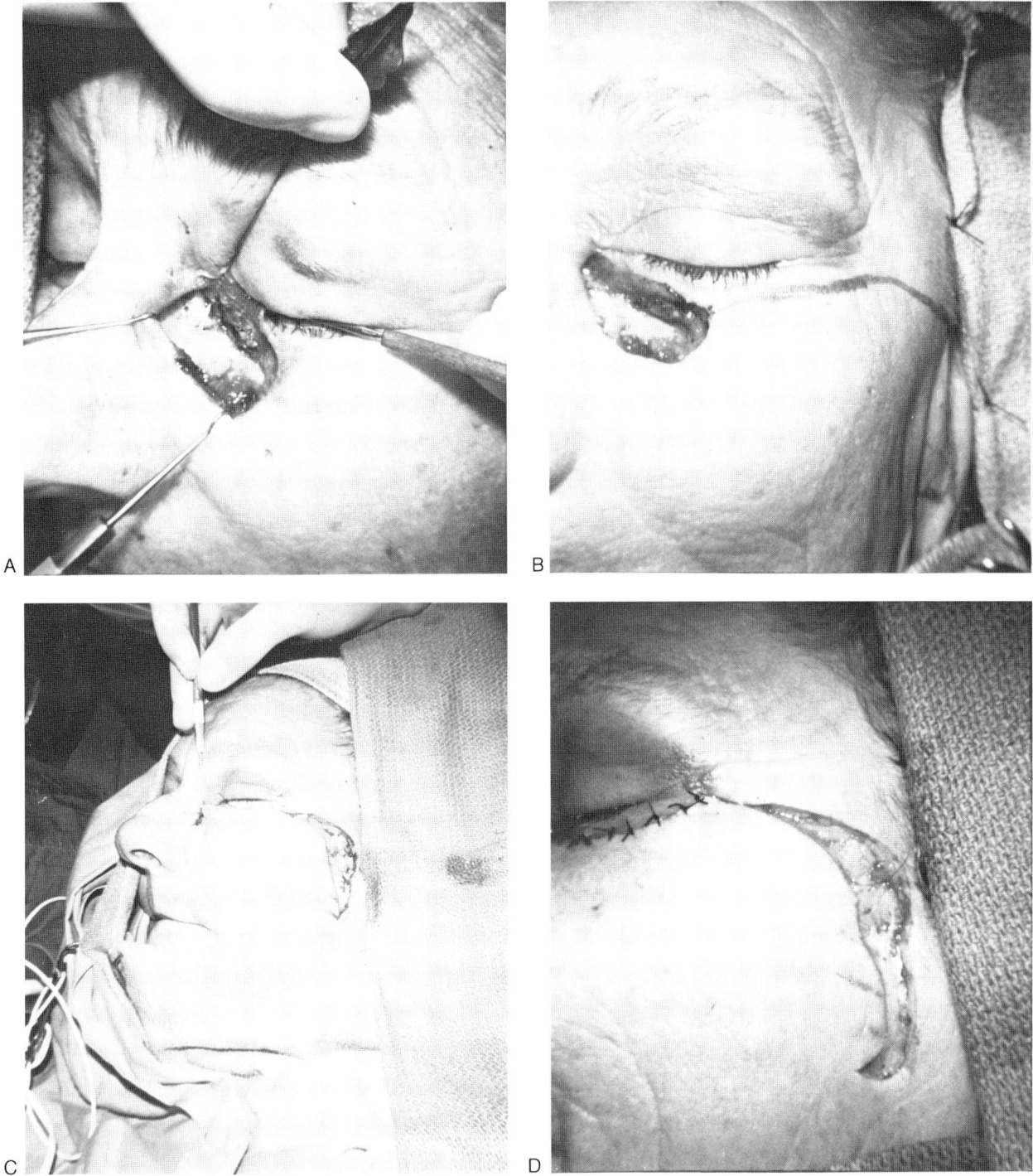

Figure 18. A, Defect created by excision of recurrent basal cell carcinoma, including lower and common canaliculi and lacrimal sac, by Mohs' technique. B, More superior location of inferiorly-based rotation cheek flap outlined. C, Flap rotated into place. D, Note back cut at base of flap.

26 Facial Reconstruction with Local and Regional Flaps

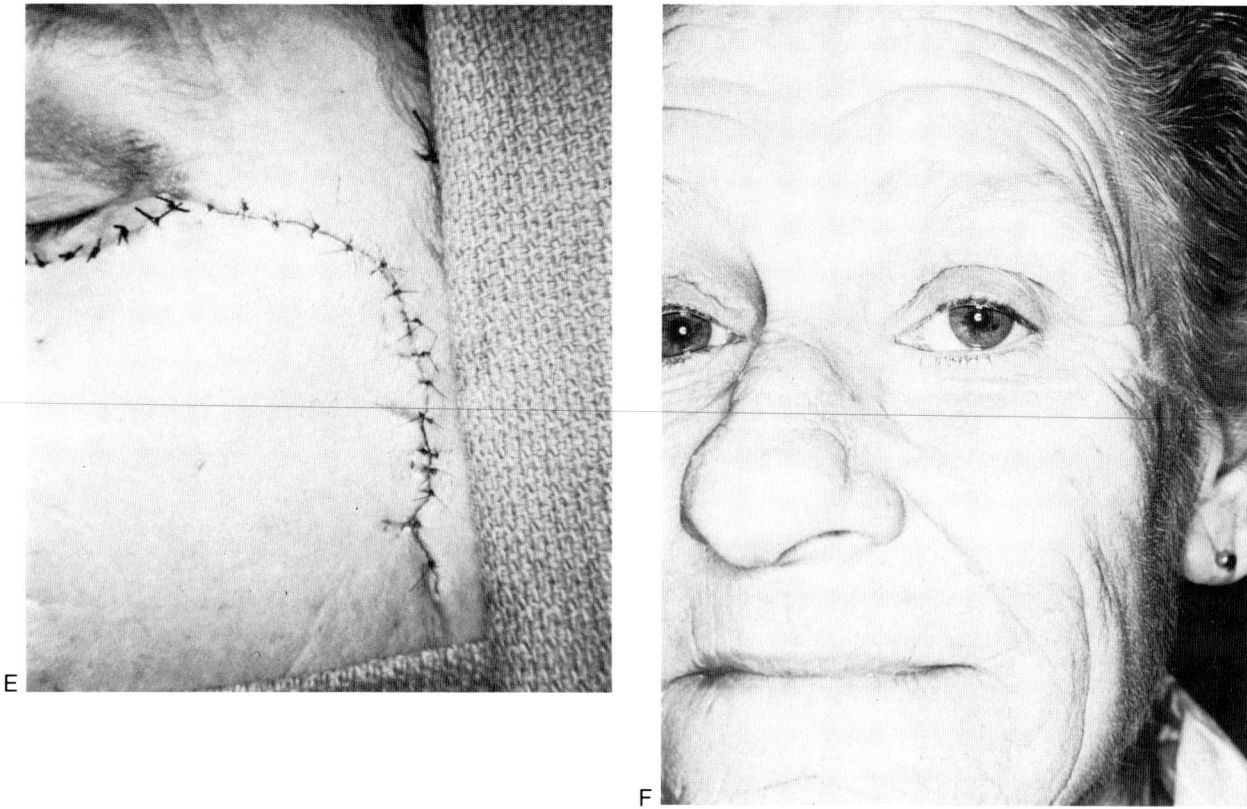

Figure 18. (cont.) E, Back cut sutured directly for closure. F, Result, 8 months postoperative.

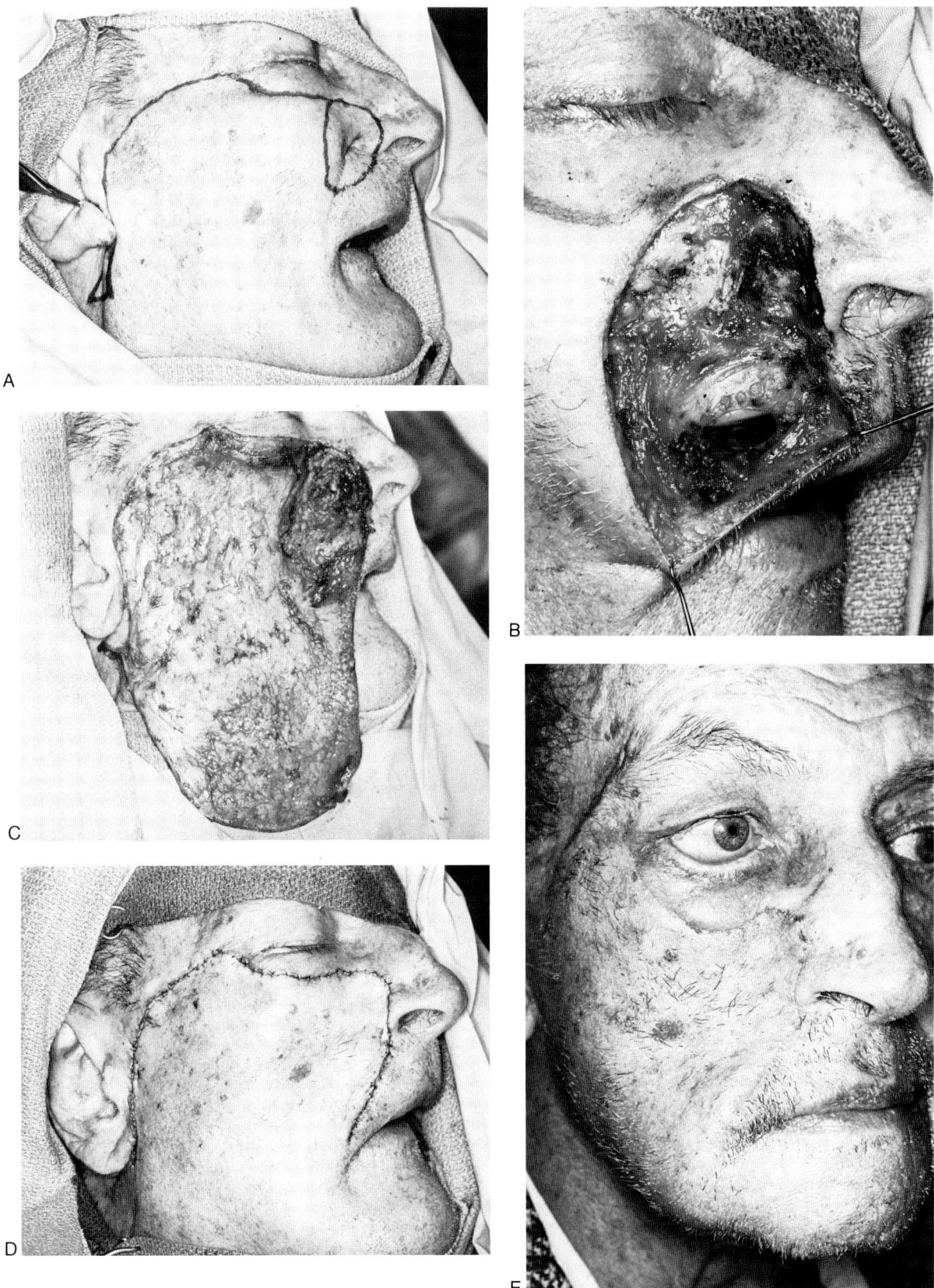

Figure 19. A, Deeply invasive recurrent basal cell carcinoma 20 years post-radiation, anteriorly-based cervicofacial flap outlined. Proposed triangle excision inferior and posterior to lobule of ear. B, Tumor excised by microscopically controlled technique of Mohs' down to bone and including the periosteum at one point. C, Flap elevated into upper neck. D, Flap rotated into place. Infra-auricular triangle closed primarily. E, Early postoperative result.

28 Facial Reconstruction with Local and Regional Flaps

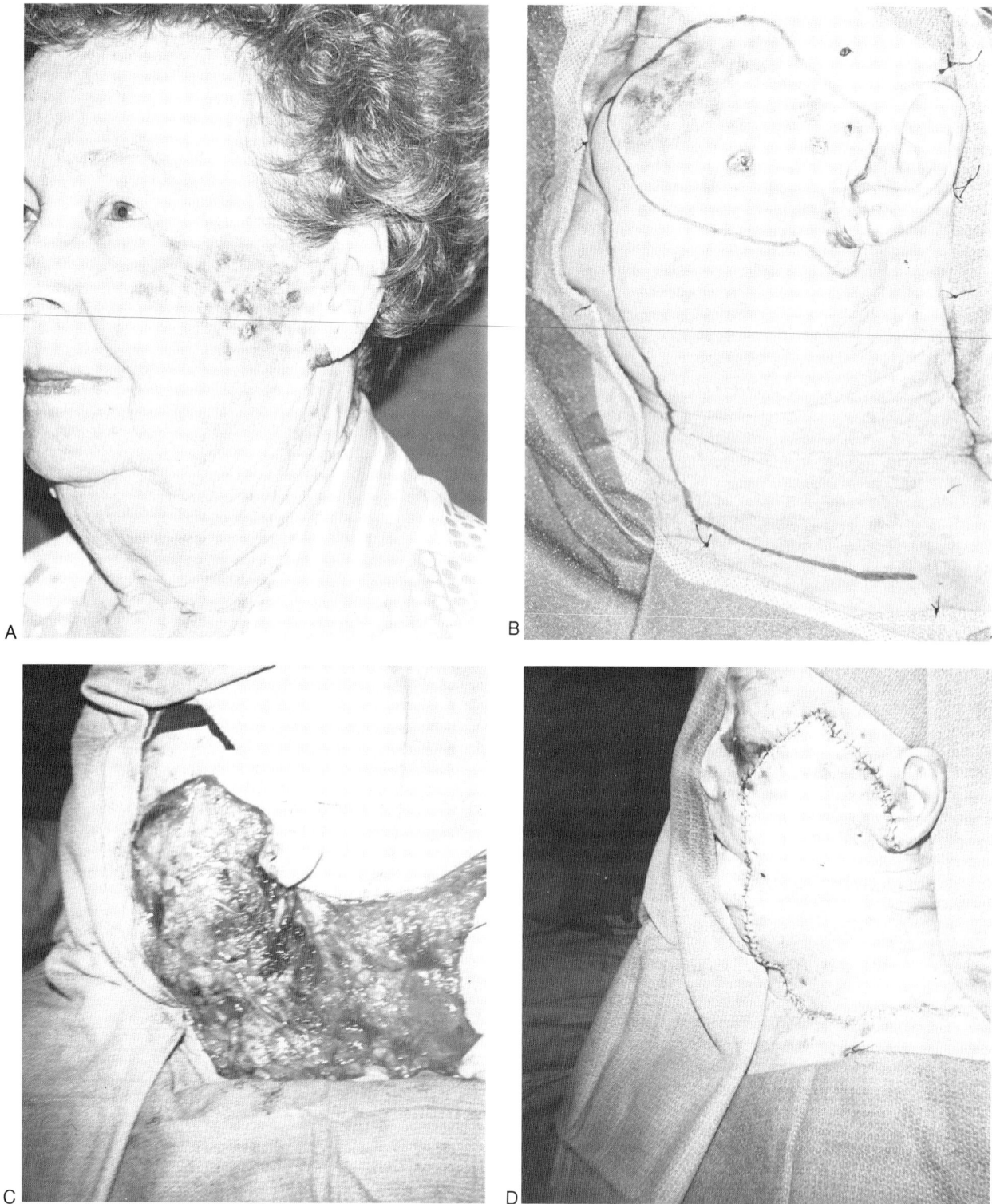

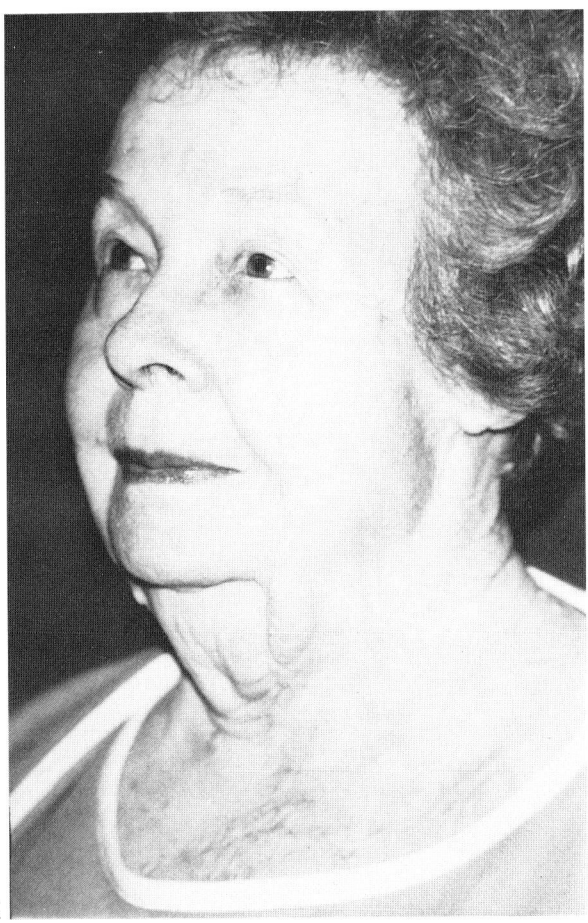

◄

Figure 20. A, Lentigo maligna melanoma of the left cheek present for ten years with areas of Level V invasion. B, Tumor excision outlined and posteriorly-based cervicofacial flap diagrammed. C, Entire cheek and left neck elevated down to clavicle. D, Flap rotated into place, donor site closed directly. E, Result, 6 months postoperative.

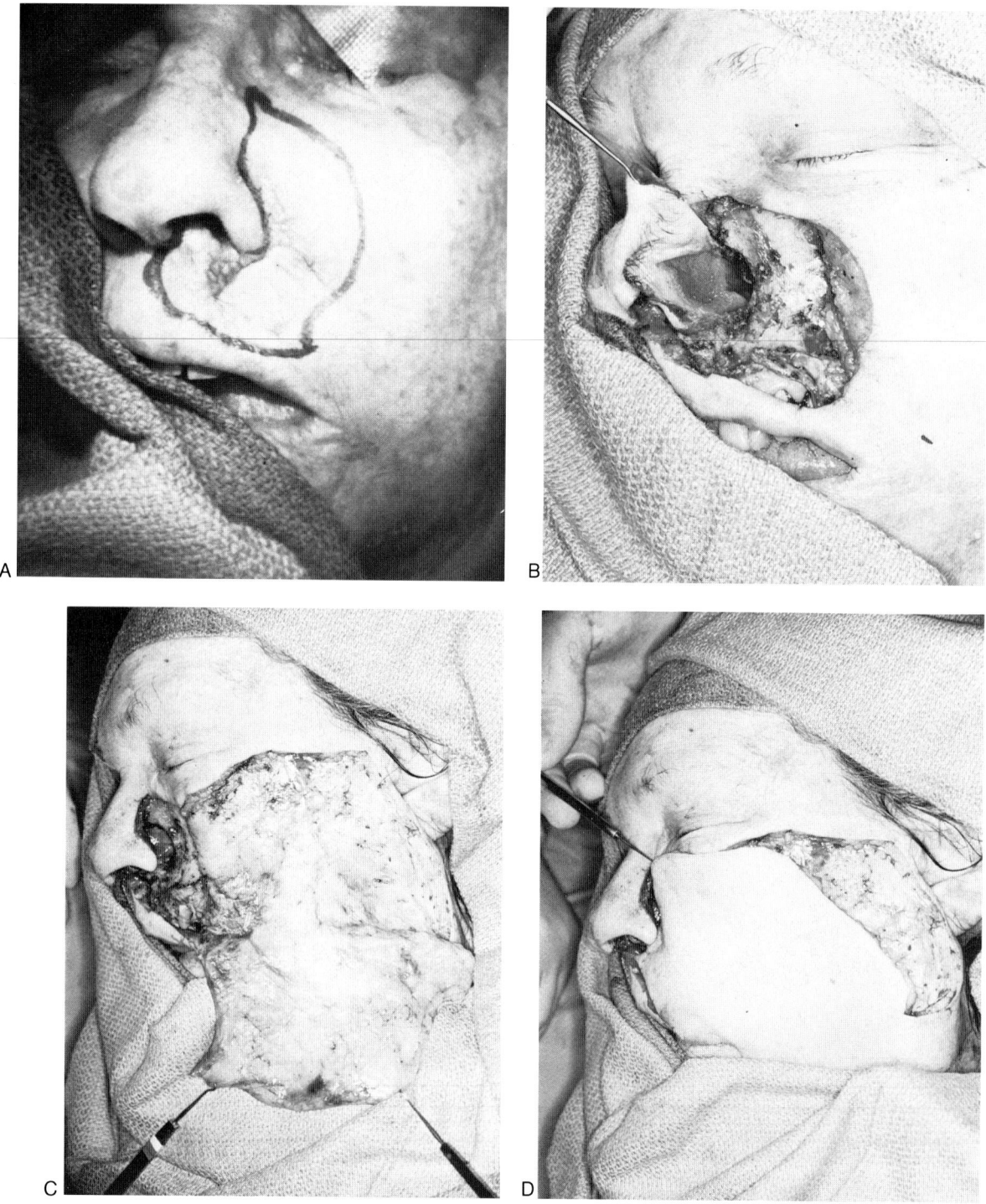

Figure 21. A, Large recurrent basal cell carcinoma after several previous attempts at removal. B, Tumor excised by microscopically controlled technique of Mohs' including upper lip, cheek, nasal ala and nose to bone. C, Large cervicofacial flap elevated. D, Flap rotated into place.

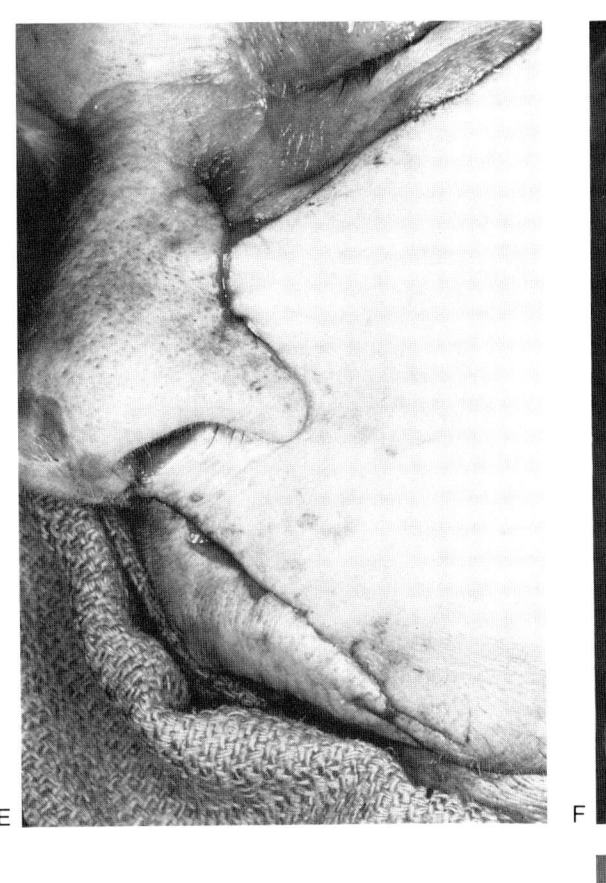
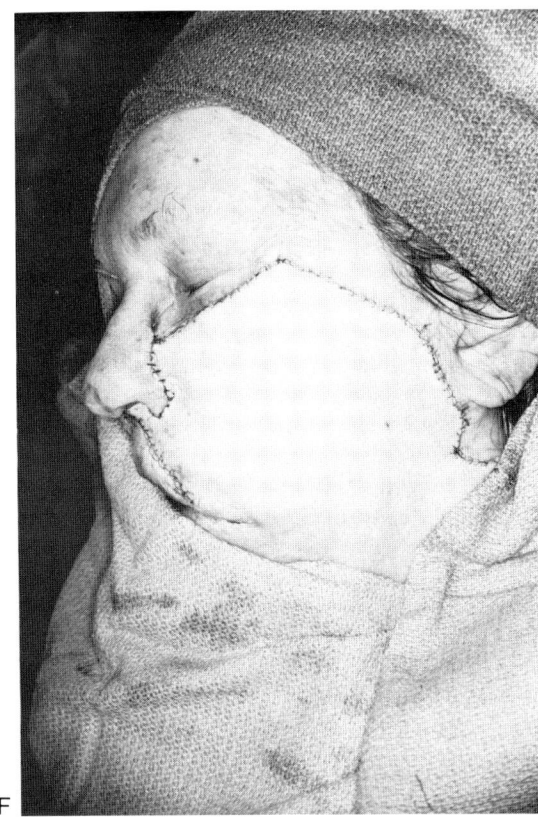
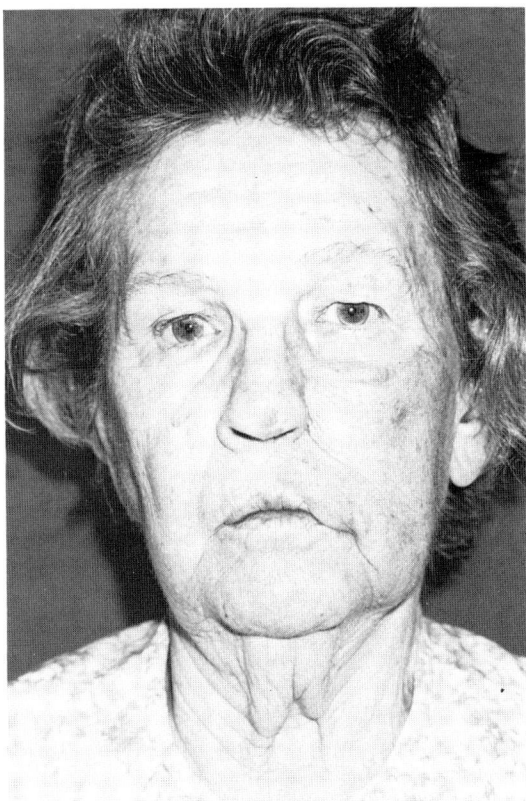

Figure 21. (cont.) E, Flap split for upper lip and nasal reconstruction. F, Final closure. G, Redundancy at rotation point of flap postoperatively.

32 Facial Reconstruction with Local and Regional Flaps

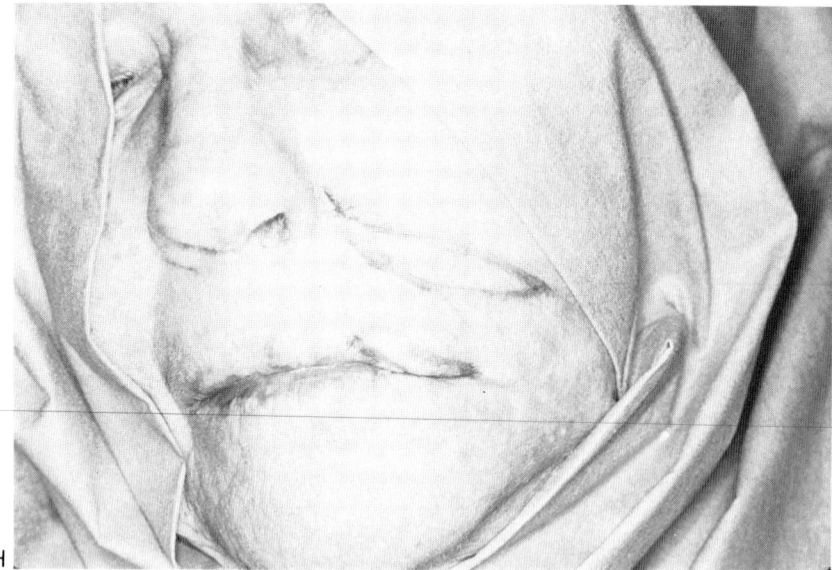

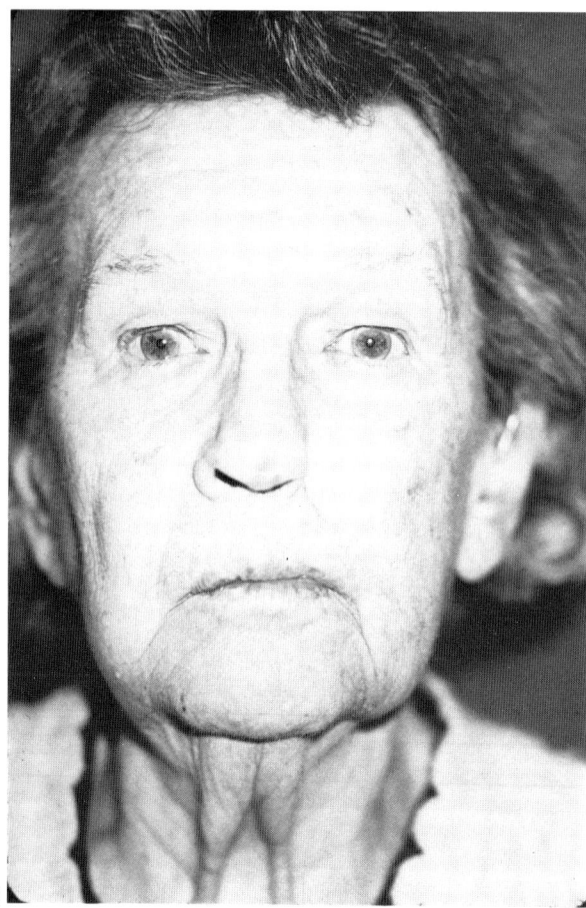

Figure 21. (cont.) H, Revision of lateral lip and nasolabial fold. I, Final result, 4 months postoperative.

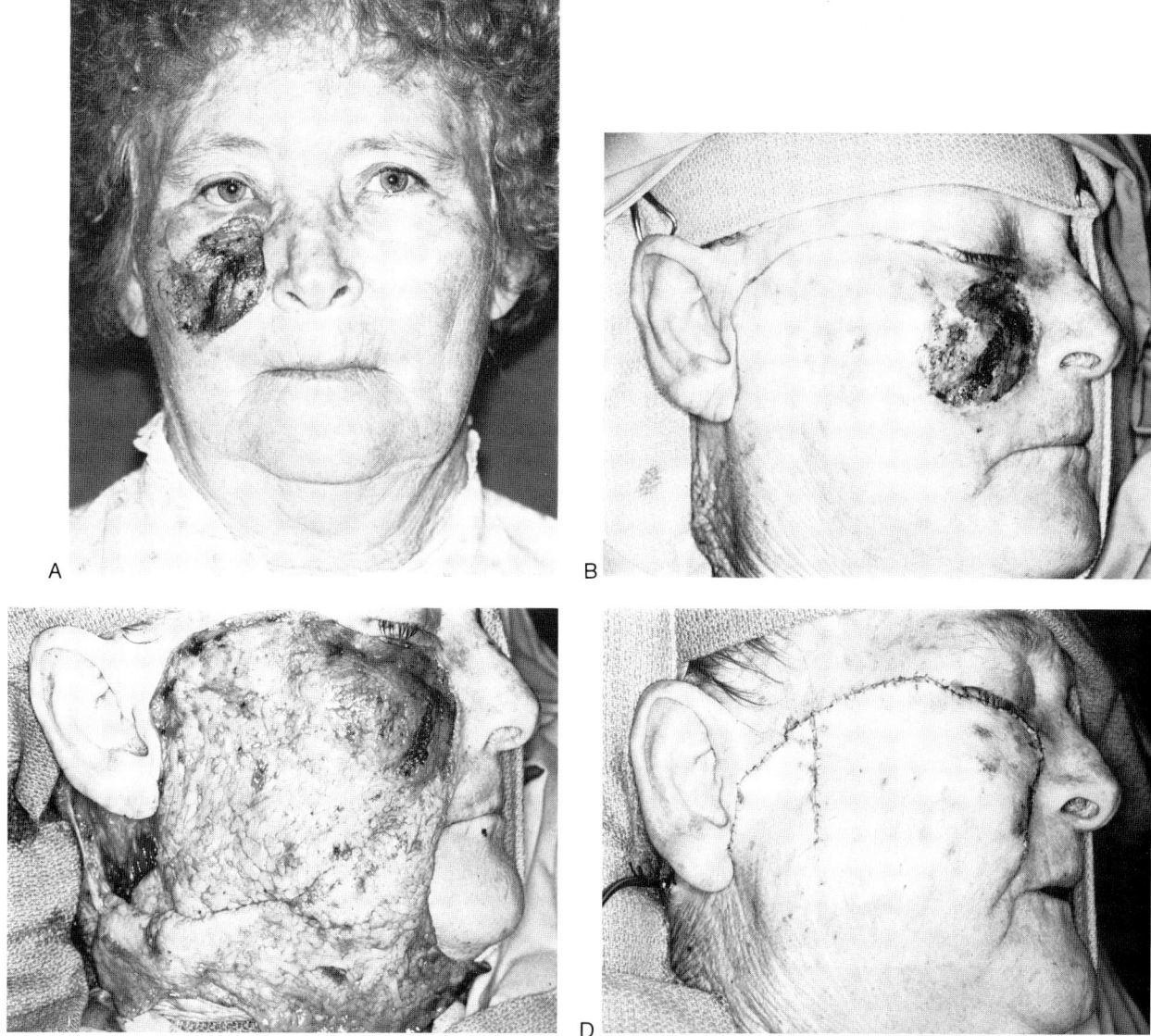

Figure 22. A, Large cheek and eyelid defect secondary to microscopically controlled excision (Mohs') of recurrent basal cell carcinoma by another Moh's surgeon. B, Cervicofacial flap outlined. C, Flap elevated with a secondary lobe posterior to the auricle. D, Flap rotated into place, second lobe rotated anterior to ear, donor site posterior to auricle closed primarily.

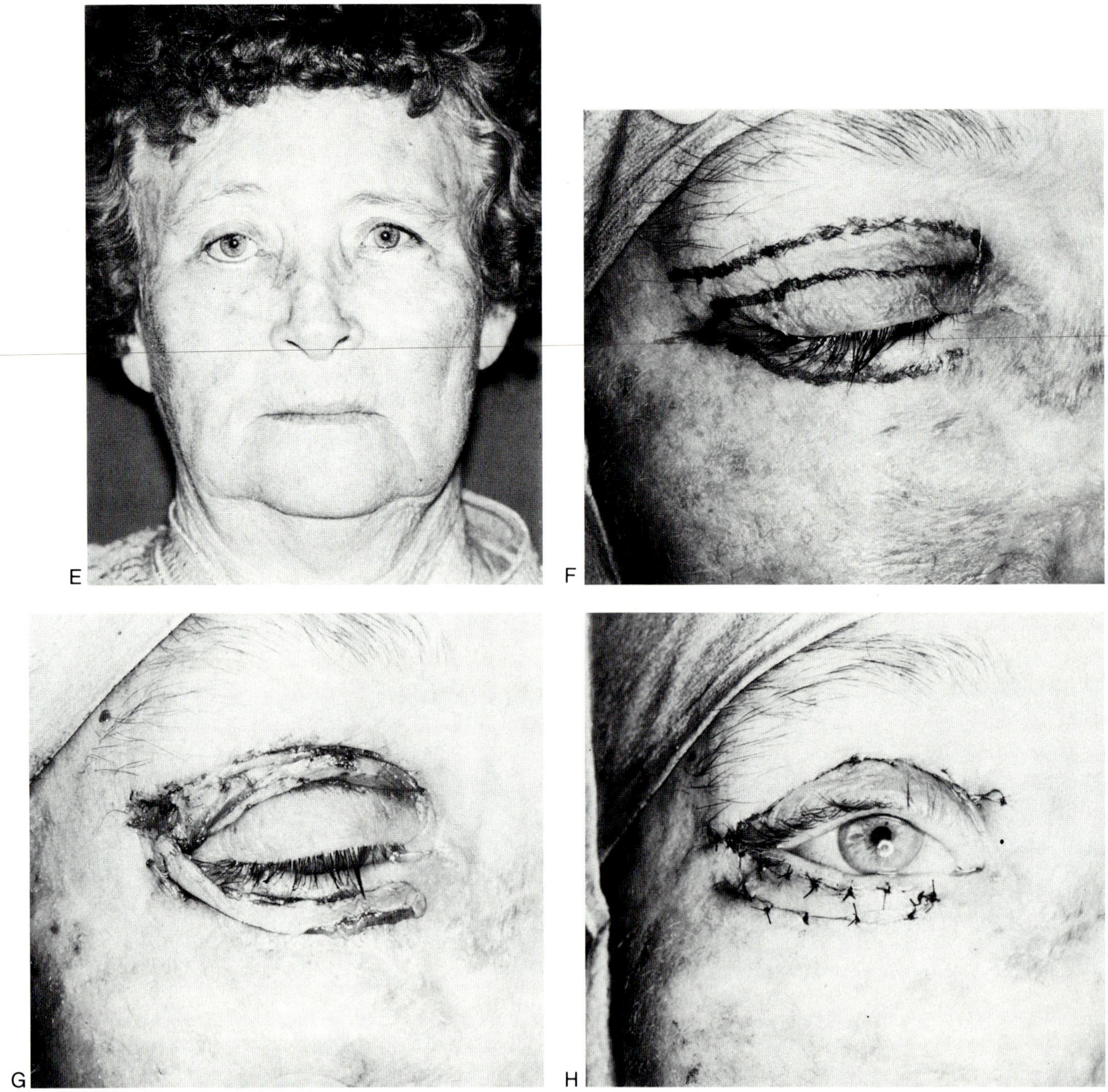

Figure 22. (cont.) E, Postoperative result with ectropion of lower eyelid. F, Laterally based upper eyelid flap outlined for correction of ectropion. G, Ectropion released, flap elevated and transposed into recipient site. H, Flap sutured into place, donor site closed in natural superior tarsal fold.

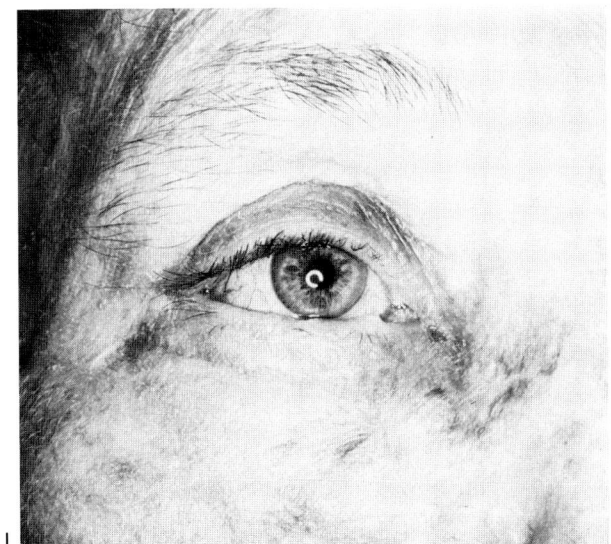 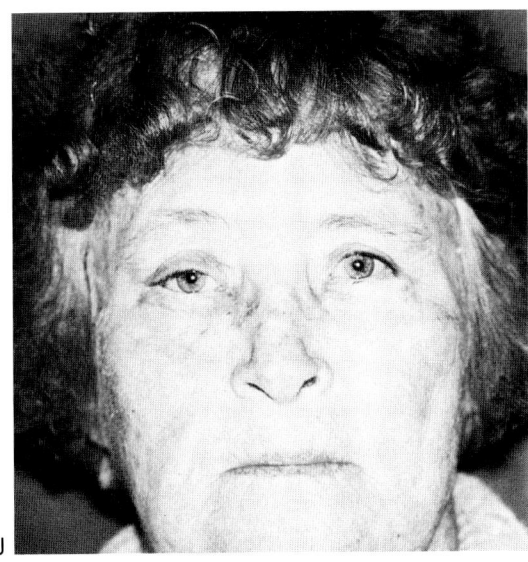

Figure 22. (cont.) I, Final postoperative result close-up. J, Final postoperative result, full face.

4 Glabellar Flaps and Dorsal Nasal Flaps

GLABELLAR FLAPS

The glabellar region is an excellent area from which to harvest adjacent skin to reconstruct defects of the superior and lateral nose, medial canthal region and even portions of the medial upper and lower eyelids. The three methods of transferring skin from the glabellar region to the upper nose and medial canthal areas are illustrated in Figure 23. Skin can be advanced directly with an advancement flap, rotated down with a V-to-Y technique or transposed over an intervening bridge of normal skin with a transposition flap. The author prefers the last approach in most glabellar flap procedures. These flaps utilize the hairless area of skin between the eyebrows and the adjacent forehead. The presence of vertical wrinkling in the glabellar area preoperatively indicates that spare skin is available for transfer and that the secondary defect can probably be closed with ease. The glabellar region is not always ideal for skin transfer. When the eyebrows meet in the midline and there is little or no hairless skin at the glabella, then it is not possible to design a flap that is devoid of hair and this method is not feasible.

The transposition glabellar flap is an excellent method for the reconstruction of medium depth defects of the medial canthal region[1] (Figure 24). The flap has an excellent color and texture match for the medial canthal skin. It can be debulked or made thicker (Figure 25) depending on the depth of the defect. The donor site is closed in a natural glabellar frownline and is often not noticeable. The primary limiting factor is the width of non-hairbearing skin in the glabellar region. It has previously been indicated[2] that the pivot point of the flap is toward the end of the flap base opposite the primary defect. In designing the flap, measurements should be taken from this point to establish whether the flap has the length to cover the defect. Generally, the flap should not extend past the medial aspect of the lower eyelid or onto the cheek. If a very large or deep medial canthal defect is present, a formal midline forehead flap might be necessary. This modality is discussed in Chapter 9.

The median glabellar flap (Figure 23A) is an advancement flap of glabellar skin down onto the superior aspect of the nose. It takes advantage of the lax skin of the glabellar region and as the tissue is advanced inferiorly, standing cones are usually excised just above the brows. The resulting short scars are not usually noticeable. Unfortunately, as McGregor[2] has pointed out, the flap causes a bridging effect at the root of the nose and tends to obscure the glabellar hollow. The angle between the nose and the brow tends to convert into the classical Greek profile. For this reason it is the author's feeling that this flap has very little use, particularly since there are better alternatives which have been discussed.

The V-to-Y glabellar flap (Figure 23B) is popular with a number of surgeons. This technique consists of a rotation of glabellar skin into a triangulated defect at the medial canthal region and lateral upper nose with closure of the donor site in a natural glabellar frownline.

DORSAL NASAL FLAPS

Rieger[3] described a technique which is essentially an extension of the V-to-Y glabellar flap onto the nose. This flap has subsequently been called the dorsal nasal flap.[4,5] It has become so popular with some authors that they have made a plea for more widespread use of this modality.[6] The flap is used for nasal tip and mid-nasal defects and consists of elevating the skin of the entire dorsum of the nose with its pedicle based on one side of the nose and with an extension into the glabellar region (Figure 26). As the skin is rotated down to fill the defect a standing cone is created at the rotation point of the flap and this must be dealt with. The skin at the inferior aspect of the flap closes the defect. This flap is essentially a V-to-Y advancement glabellar flap combined with a nasal rotation flap as pointed out by Cronin.[7] This flap has been found useful for outer covering of a full thickness lower nasal defect (Figure 27). While it is a very useful flap, this rather elaborate technique should probably not be used when a simpler technique for nasal tip reconstruction would give a similar or superior result.

REFERENCES

1. Becker FF: Reconstructive surgery of the medial canthal region. Ann Plast Surg 7:259–268, 1981
2. McGregor IA: Local skin flaps in facial reconstruction. Otolaryngol Clin NA 15:77–98, 1982
3. Rieger RA: A local flap for repair of the nasal tip. Plast Reconstr Surg 49:147, 1967
4. Rigg BM: The dorsal nasal flap. Plast Reconstr Surg 52:361, 1973
5. Avahoff JC: The dorsal nasal flap. Plast Reconstr Surg 53:671, 1974
6. Bray DA, Eichel BS, Kaplan HJ: The dorsal nasal flap. Arch Otolaryngol 107:765–766, 1981
7. Cronin TD: The V-Y rotational flap for nasal tip defects. Ann Plast Surg 11:282–288, 1983

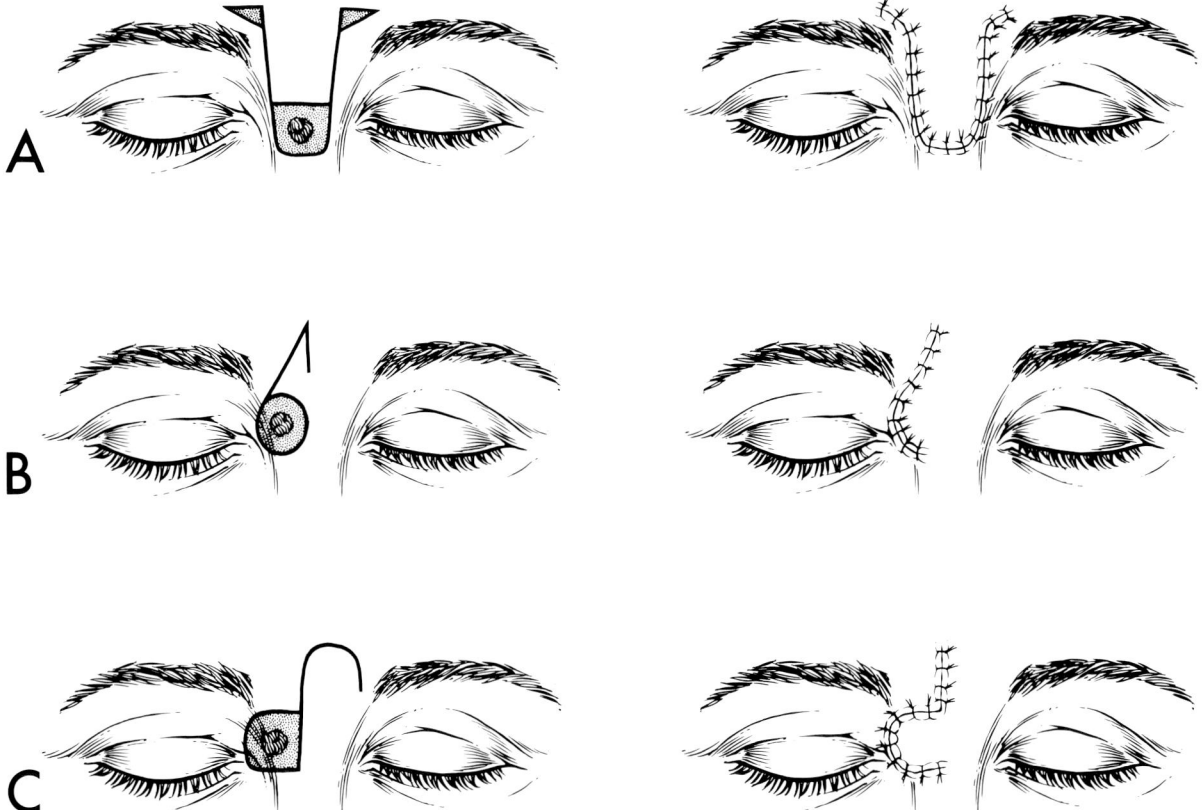

Figure 23. Types of Glabellar Flaps. A, Advancement glabellar flap; note triangles of skin to be removed above medial brows. B, V-to-Y rotation glabellar flap. C, Transposition glabellar flap.

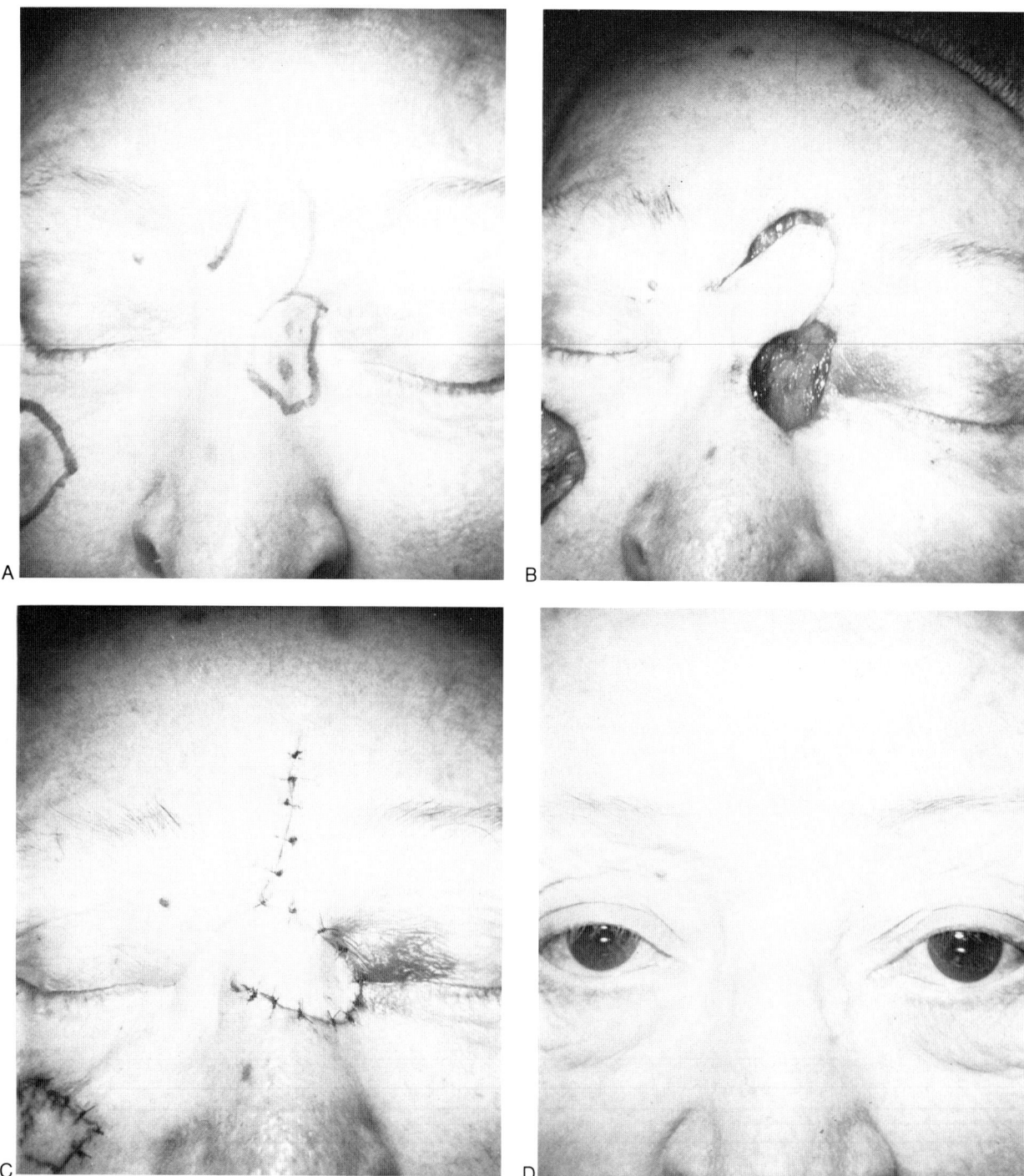

Figure 24. A, Two basal cell carcinomas outlined for removal in medial canthal region, glabellar flap outlined. B, Tumor excised, flap incised and elevated. C, Flap transposed into place, donor site closed in natural glabellar frown line. D, Final postoperative result.

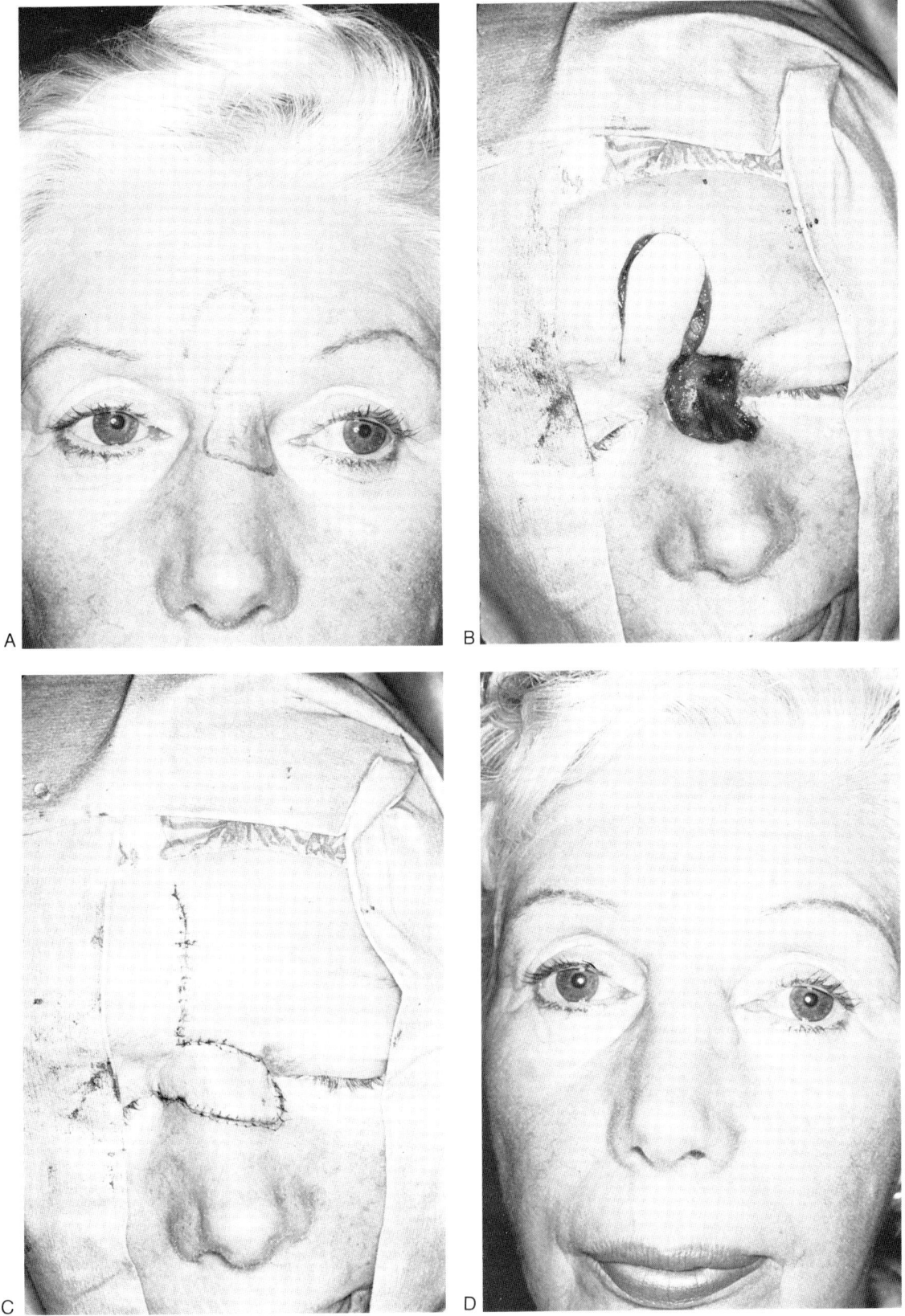

Figure 25. A, Recurrent basal cell carcinoma of nasal dorsum outlined, glabellar flap designed. B, Tumor excised to periosteum by Mohs' technique, flap elevated. C, Flap rotated into place. D, Final result, one year postoperative.

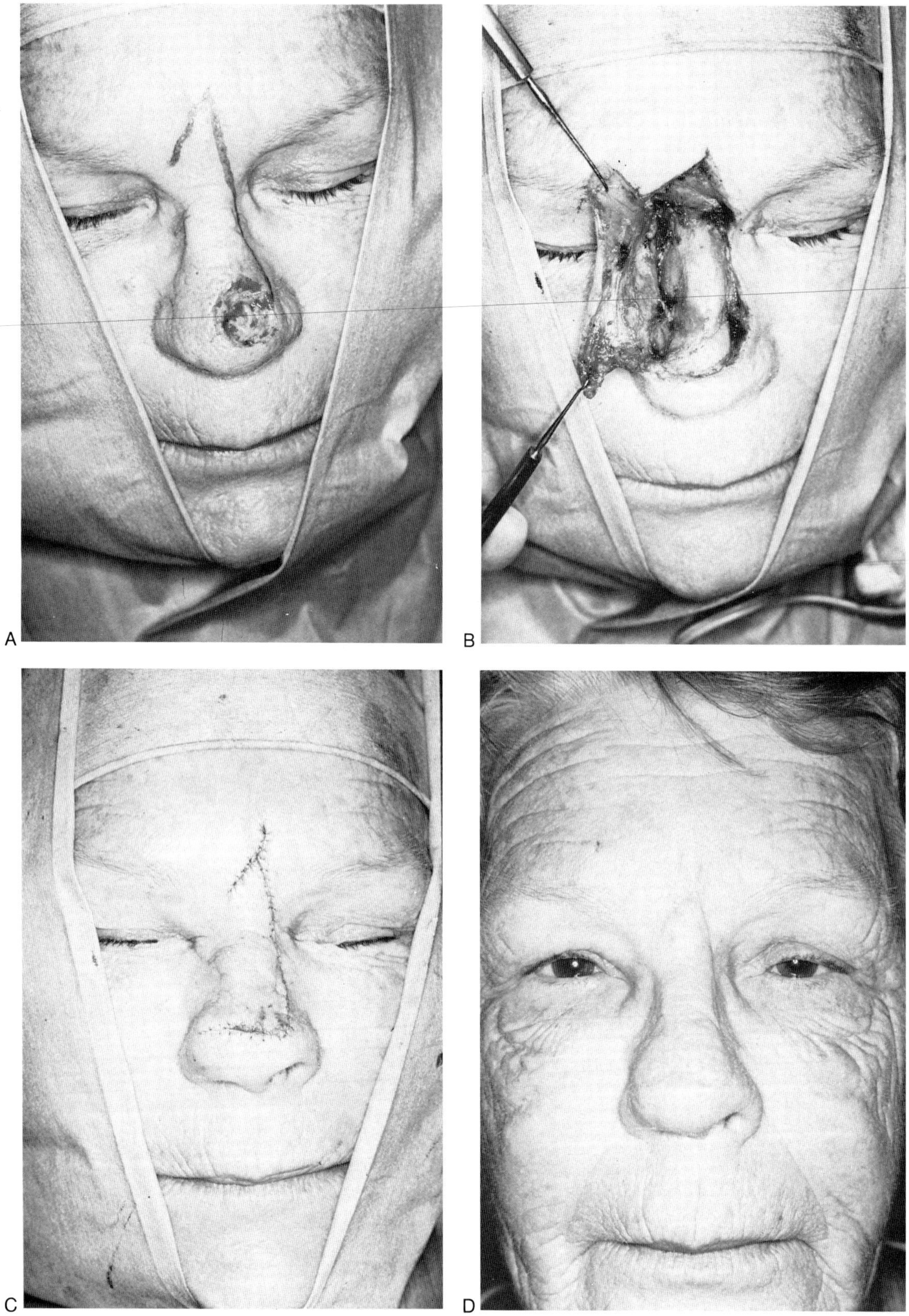

Figure 26. A, Tumor excised, dorsal nasal flap outlined. B, Flap elevated in plane superficial to periosteum and perichondrium of nasal dorsum. C, Flap rotated into place with donor site closed directly in a V-to-Y manner at glabella. D, Postoperative result.

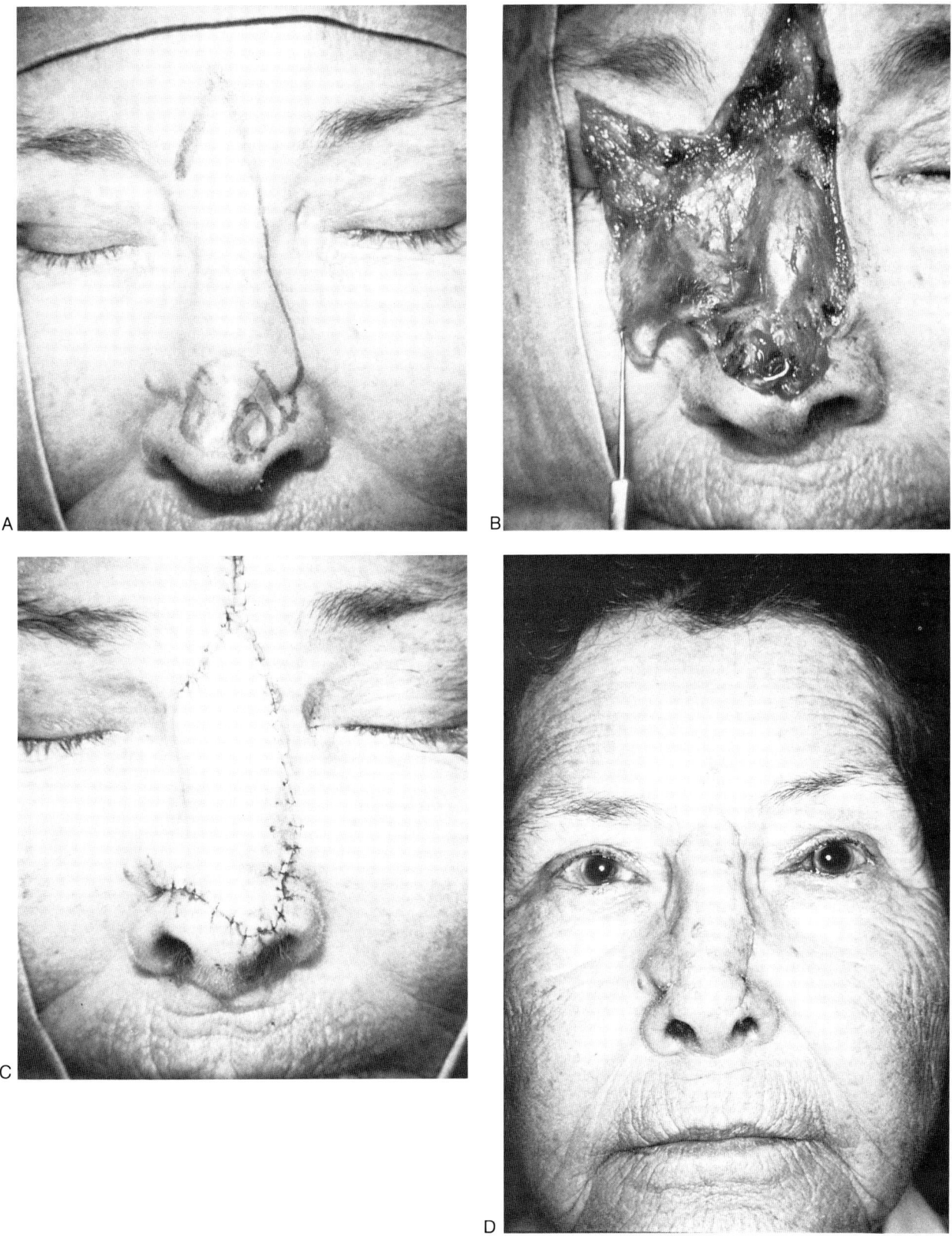

Figure 27. A, Tumor excision and dorsal nasal flap outlined. B, Tumor excised with small through and through defect, flap elevated. C, Flap in place, donor site closed in V-to-Y manner. D, Postoperative result.

5 Rhombic Flaps

Since Limberg's classical description of his flap in 1946,[1] there has been an enormous interest in this subject in the literature. Dufourmentel[2] and Webster[3] have described well recognized modifications of Limberg's classical design. Multiple rhomboid flap closures, rhomboid to W techniques[4] and many other variations have also been described. The geometry of all these concepts is appealing but the more compound and complex the flaps are made, the worse the scarring that results. This flap of Limberg and the modification of Dufourmentel should be studied and mastered, and will suffice in most cases where these flaps are applicable. In order to avoid using an eponym, the flap had been termed the rhomboid flap for several years. Borges[5] pointed out that the defect being closed is a rhombus and not a rhomboid, and therefore the flap should be called the rhombic flap. The author, as well as others,[6] has chosen to adhere to this terminology. Dufourmentel's modification would be the modified rhombic flap.

It would appear that one of the most appealing aspects of the rhombic flap is its precise geometric design. Figure 28 illustrates the design of the basic rhombic flap and its transfer as well as its major modifications. It can be seen from this figure that the rhombus is an equilateral parallelogram with oblique angles. The classic angles are 60° and 120°, but this can vary slightly. The rhombus is drawn around the proposed area of excision. A line is drawn perpendicularly from one side of the rhombus and is of equal length with its sides. Another limb is drawn at a 60° angle from the end of this line in either direction. After the defect is created, the flap is raised and transposed into the defect (point 6 moves closer to point 4), thereby partially closing the donor defect. The author pointed out in 1979[7] that the line of maximum tension on this flap is at the closure point of the donor flap defect (point 4–6). In fact, if the flap and tissue surrounding the rhombic defect are adequately undermined, and the donor site is closed completely, there should be little or no tension on the end of the flap (point 2–8) after it has been transposed (Figure 29). The Dufourmentel modification (Figure 34) makes closure of the donor site easier and is an important contribution. With this modification, it must be remembered that even after closure of the donor site, some of the tension is shared by the tissue adjacent to the defect since the flap is somewhat more narrow than the classical rhombic flap.

Borges[5] described a simplified method for designing and orienting this flap for routine use. This technique is illustrated in Figure 30. First, a clear understanding of the relaxed skin tension lines (RSTL) must be firmly imprinted in the mind of the surgeon. The lines of maximum extensibility (LME) run perpendicular to the RSTL. Readers are referred to another work of Borges[8] for excellent diagrams and illustrations on that subject. Two parallel lines are drawn following the LME and tangential to the tissue to be excised. Two other lines are drawn to complete the rhombus with 60° and 120° angles. Two umbrella-like designs are drawn with each stem drawn as an extension of the short diagonal of the rhombic defect and the other limbs parallel to one of its sides. Four possible donor rhombic flaps are thus formed. Choosing a rhombic flap with its short diagonal following the LME is crucial. This is the only way to take full advantage of the difference in tension between the LME and the RSTL. The well chosen rhombic flap actually pulls skin from where it is plentiful (following the LME). Clinically, it usually is quite obvious that the umbrella on one side of the rhombic defect is an unsuitable area and that the correct flap must be chosen from the opposite side. On the opposite side there is only one rhombic flap with the closure point of its donor site in an LME and this is usually the correct flap to choose. Figure 31 is a case of a correctly oriented rhombic flap. It is the author's view that Borges' method of designing and orienting the flap is entirely correct and should be adhered to with one very important exception, as pointed out previously.[7] The surgeon must be careful to plan the flap so that the final line of tension (the line of closure of the donor site) is oriented in such a way that it does not distort a prominent landmark of the face, such as a nasal ala, a canthus, an eyelid, a brow or the oral commissure. Figure 32 shows a case in which the flap was oriented correctly by the Borges technique. However, the tension on the line of closure of the donor site caused a considerable pull on the lateral commissure of the mouth. One year postoperatively this had loosened up, but it could have been avoided if the flap had been designed differently. Figure 33 shows a case in which the flap was designed so that the closure of the donor site did not cause tension on the lower eyelid and therefore an ectropion was avoided. The Dufourmentel modification is quite helpful since there is less tension on the closure line. Figure 34 shows a modified rhombic flap that worked quite nicely even though it was not designed according to the Borges principle.

In a series of 30 rhombic flaps studied previously,[7] it was found that the anatomical areas most useful for the rhombic flap were the cheeks, temples and nose in that order. It was also felt that the results obtained were far superior to those which could have been achieved with skin grafts in most cases. The cases were critically analyzed for results and complications. In cases in which great tension was exerted to close the donor site, a slight depression along this line of tension (closure) was noted in some cases. Although this tended to resolve with time, if this depression was over a bony landmark (nose, mandible) it could be more noticeable. Of six cases in which the line of maximum tension crossed a bony prominence, only one showed any permanent depression. No other significant complications were noted in that series.

The author would like to join Dr. Borges in making a plea for simplicity in the design and execution of the rhombic flap. While the multiple rhombic flap procedures are appealing geometrically, it is the author's feeling that practical application of those techniques is very limited and that increased scarring will result. The classical rhombic flap or its primary modification is usually all that is necessary, and a thorough understanding of the principles of design and execution of the flaps which have been discussed in this chapter can be easily mastered and successfully used for reconstruction of many facial defects.

REFERENCES

1. Limberg AA: Mathematical Principles of Local Plastic Procedures of the Surface of the Human Body. Leningrad: Medgiz, 1946
2. Dufourmentel C: Le formeture des portes de substance cutance limitees "le labeaude rotation on 1 pour losarge "dit LLL". Ann Chir Plast 7:61–66, 1962
3. Webster RC, Davidson TM, Smith RC: The thirty degree transposition flap. Laryngoscope 88:85–94, 1978
4. Becker H: The rhomboid-to-W technique for excision of some skin lesions and closure. Plast Reconstr Surg 64:444, 1979
5. Borges AF: The rhombic flap. Plast Reconstr Surg 67:458, 1981
6. Gunter JR: Rhombic flaps. Facial Plast Surg 1:69–73, 1983
7. Becker FF: Rhomboid flap in facial reconstruction: new concept of tension lines. Arch Otolaryngol 105:569–573, 1979
8. Borges AF: Elective Incisions and Scar Revisions. Boston: Little Brown & Co, 1973

Figure 28. A, Design of rhombic flap (Limberg). B, A completed rhombic flap showing the line of maximum tension at closure of donor site. C, Modified rhombic flap (Dufourmentel): Angle 4–5–6 is made less than 60°. This decreases the width of the flap and makes closure of the donor site easier. It must be remembered that this modification makes the flap slightly smaller than the defect and therefore tension must be shared by the edges of the defect. D, 30° transposition flap (Webster): This makes an even more narrow angle at 4–5–6; the base of this flap is also narrowed considerably.

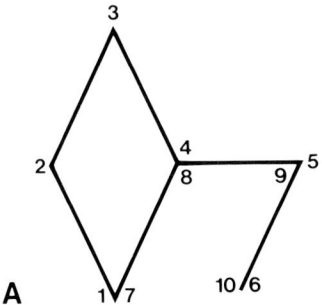
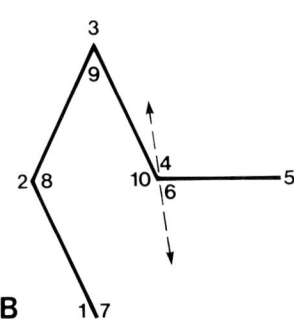
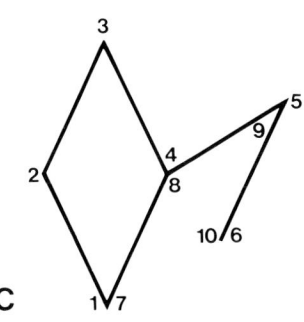
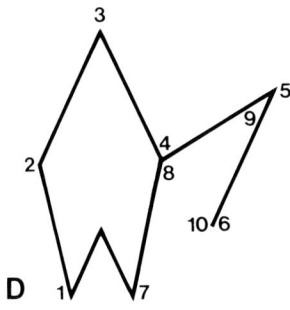

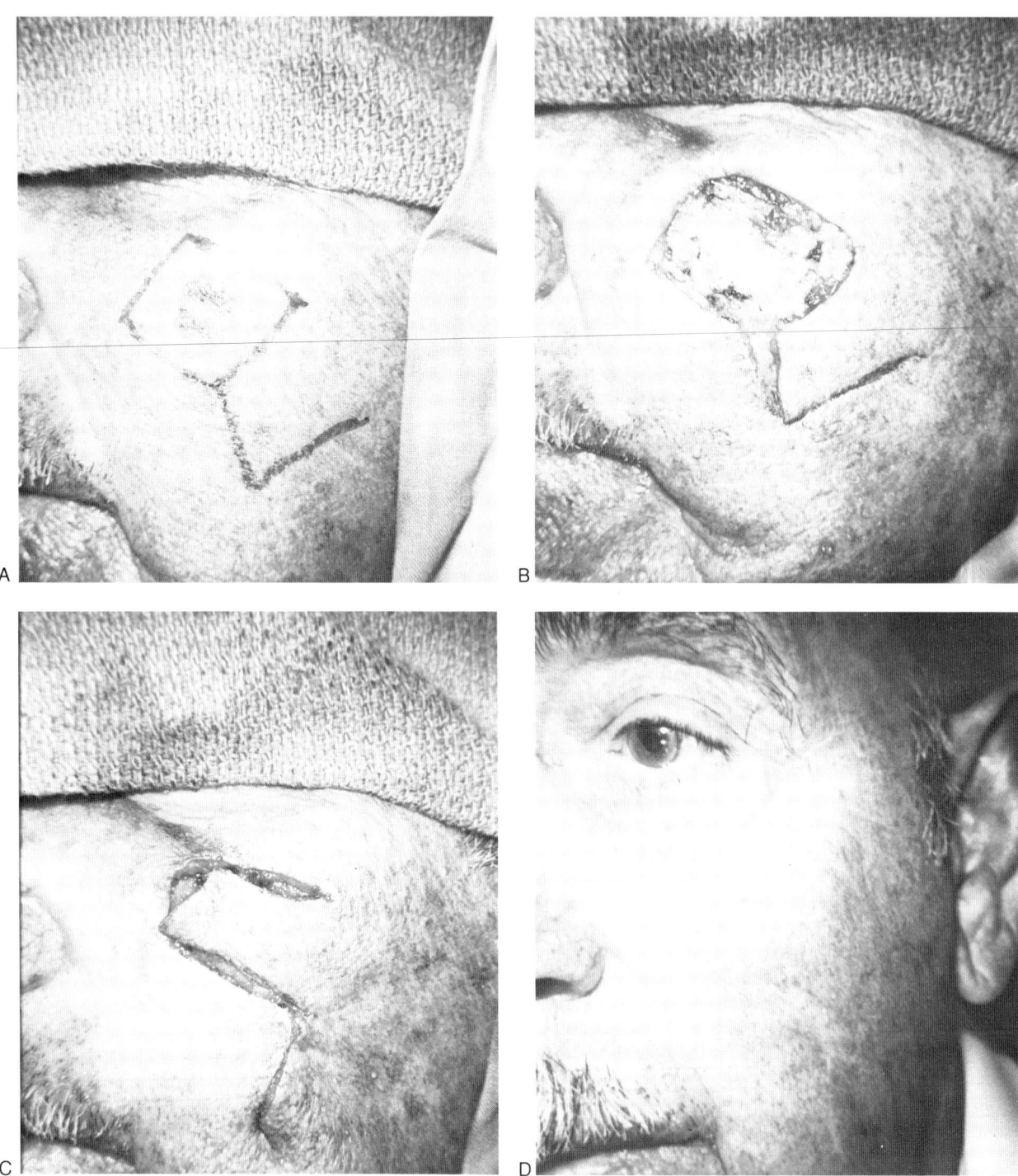

Figure 29. A, Lentigo maligna of left cheek, rhombic flap outlined. B, Tumor removed, flap elevated. C, Flap rotated into place, one subcutaneous suture closing donor site at line of maximum tension, which is located in a LME; virtually no tension on the end of flap that is unsutured. D, Final result, one year postoperative. (Reprinted with permission from: Becker FF: Rhomboid flap in facial reconstruction. Arch Otolaryngol 105:569–573, 1979. Copyright 1979, American Medical Association)

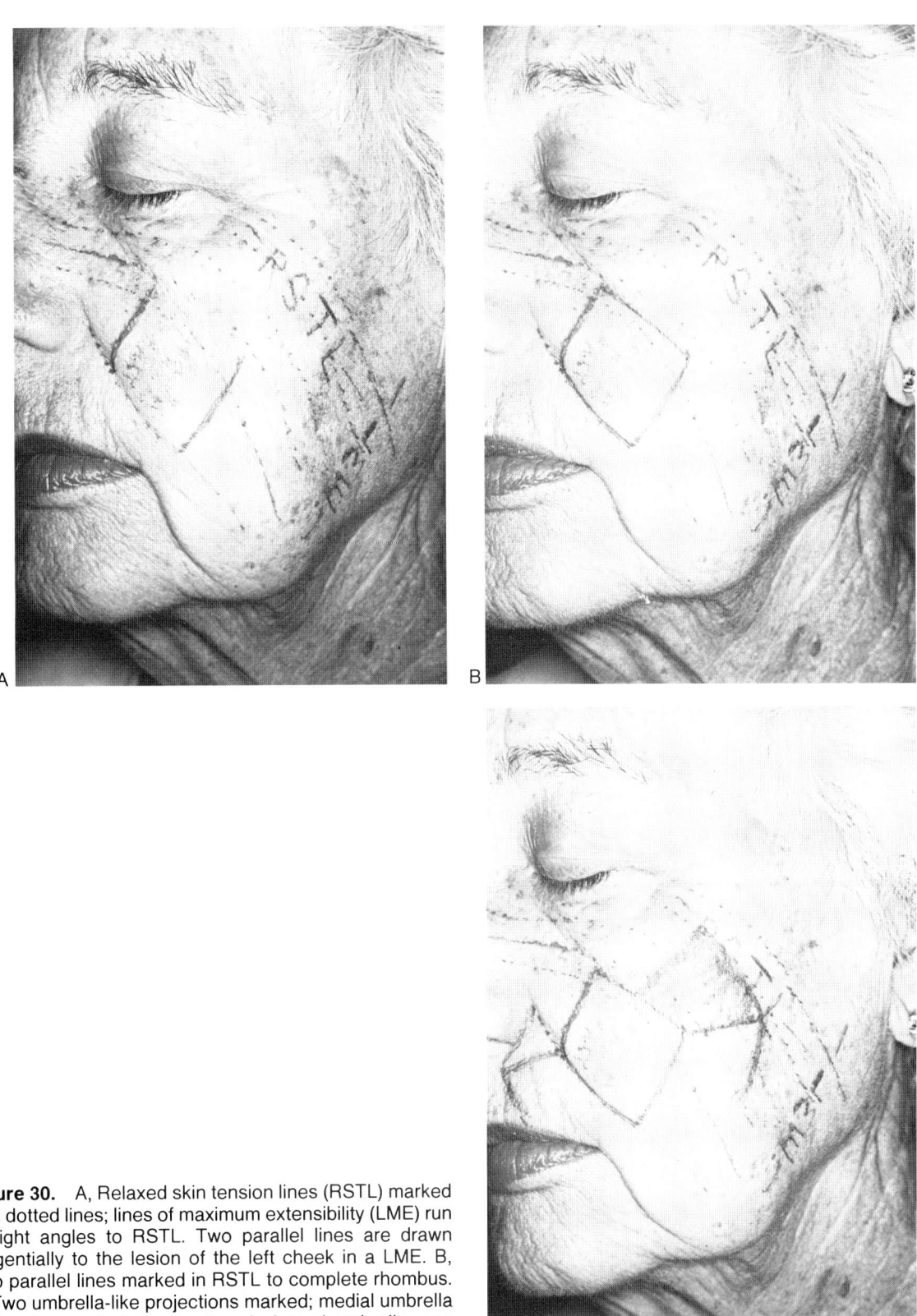

Figure 30. A, Relaxed skin tension lines (RSTL) marked with dotted lines; lines of maximum extensibility (LME) run at right angles to RSTL. Two parallel lines are drawn tangentially to the lesion of the left cheek in a LME. B, Two parallel lines marked in RSTL to complete rhombus. C, Two umbrella-like projections marked; medial umbrella obviously unsuited for any flap. In lateral umbrella, one flap (shaded) will leave the line of maximum tension (closure of donor site) in a LME.

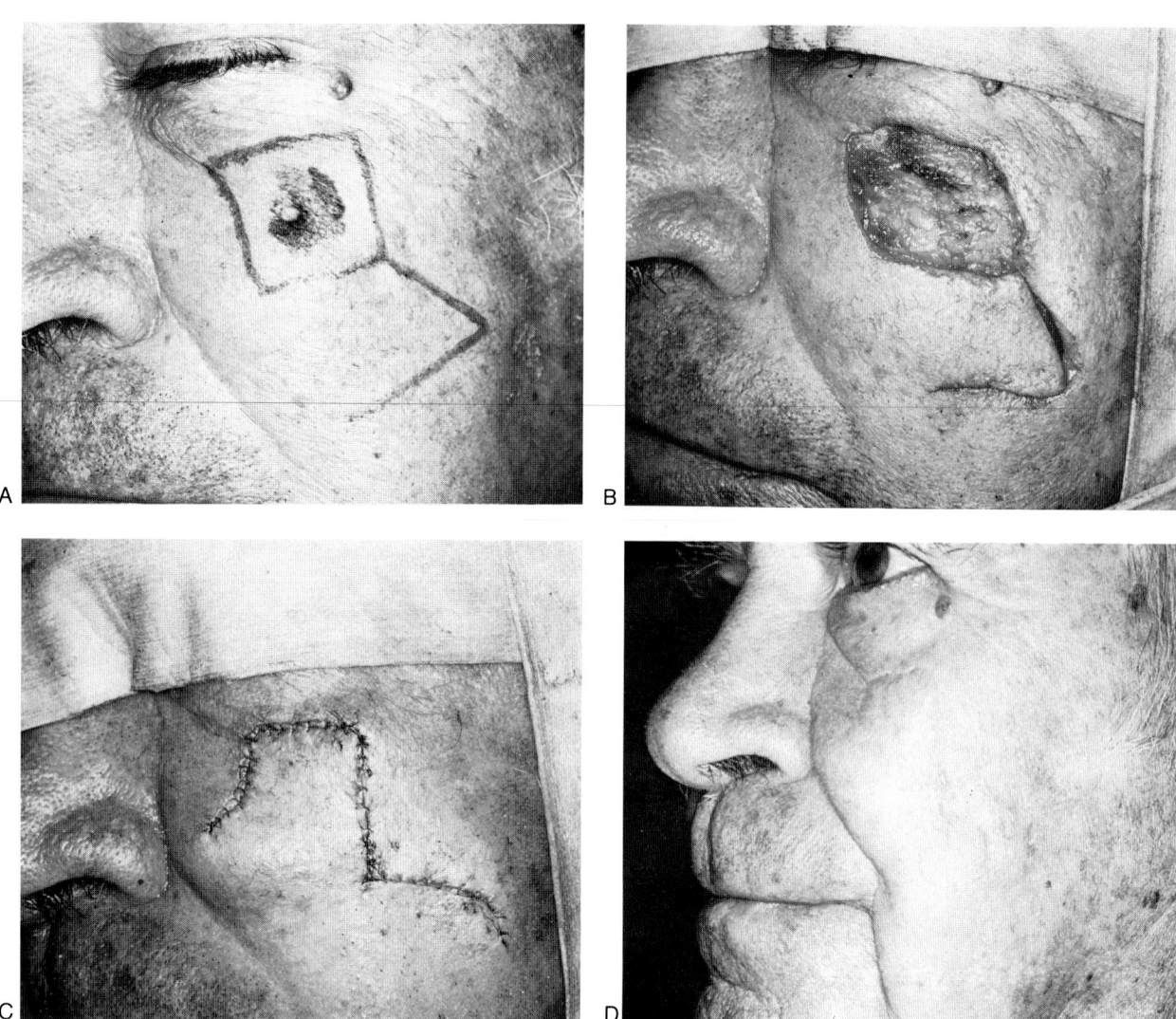

Figure 31. A, Excision surrounding lentigo maligna of left cheek marked with rhombus; rhombic flap marked with line of closure corresponding to a LEM. B, Tumor excised, flap elevated. C, Flap rotated into place. D, Final result, 8 months postoperative.

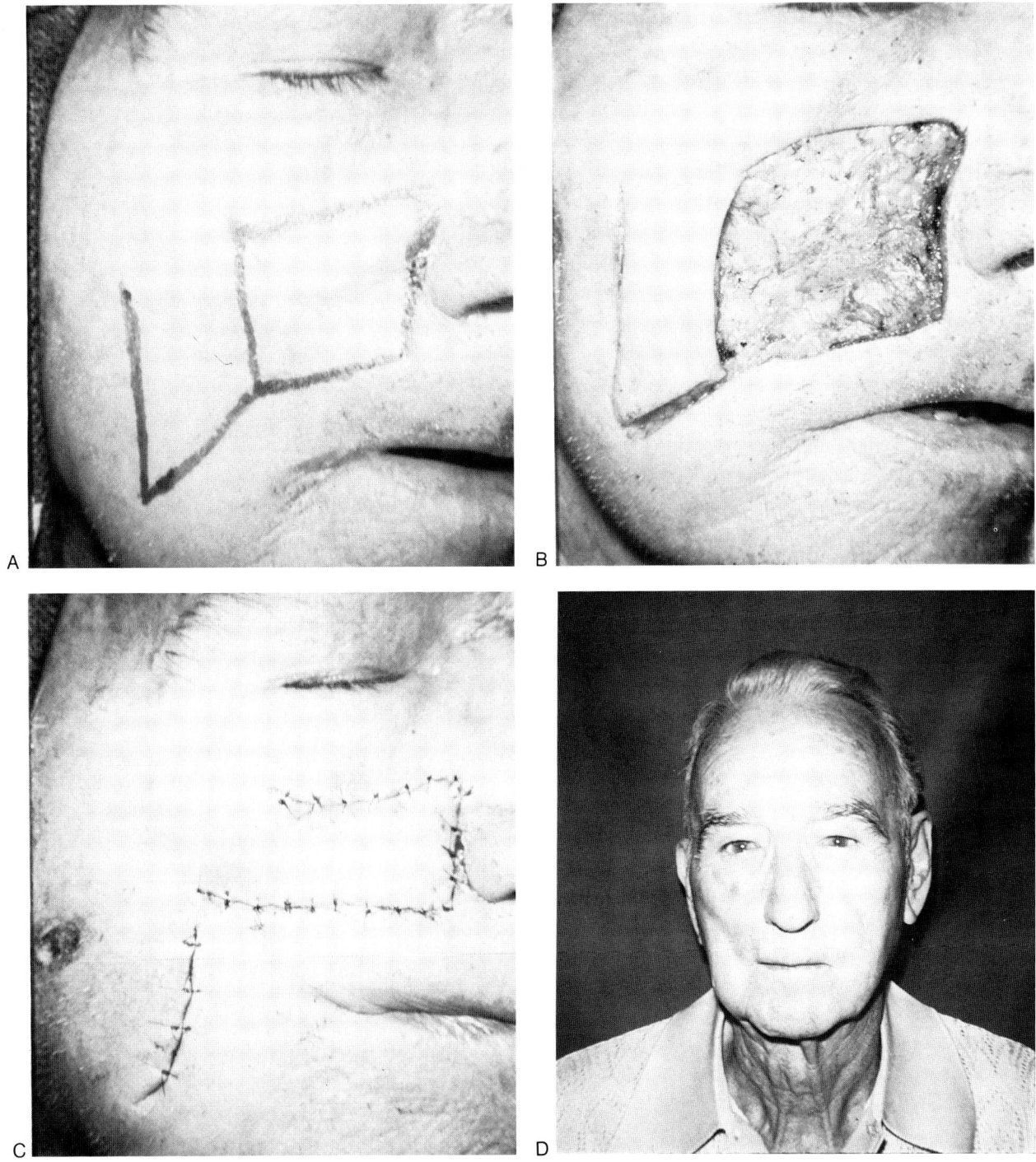

Figure 32. A, Rhombus outlined for excision of residual lentigo maligna melanoma of cheek. Flap outlined with closure of donor site in a LME. However, the line of maximum tension is located at the lateral commissure of the mouth. B, Tumor excised, flap elevated. C, Flap rotated into place. Note extreme tension on lateral commissure of the mouth. D, Final result, one year postoperative. Distortion is not noted now, but was prior to this time. (Reprinted with permission from: Becker FF: Rhomboid flap in facial reconstruction. Arch Otolaryngol 105:569–573, 1979. Copyright 1979, American Medical Association)

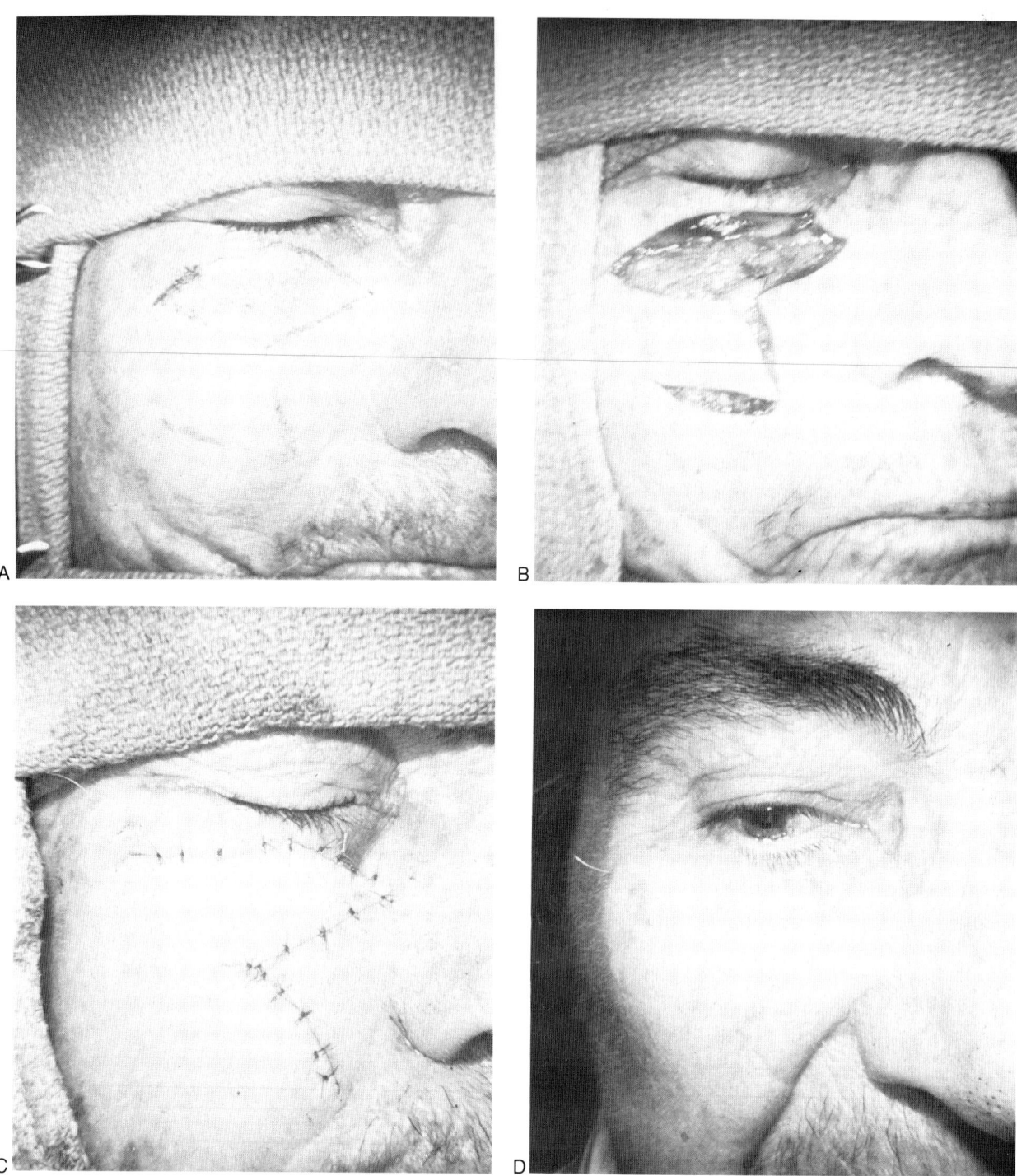

Figure 33. A, Excision of large diffuse basal cell carcinoma of lower eyelid and cheek outlined in rhombus design, and flap outline with proposed closure site in a relaxed skin tension line. However, there should be no pull on lower eyelid. B, Tumor excised, flap elevated. C, Flap rotated into place, donor site closed. D, Final result, one year postoperative. Note: no pull on lower eyelid. (Reprinted with permission from: Becker FF: Rhomboid flap in facial reconstruction. Arch Otolaryngol 105:569–573, 1979. Copyright 1979, American Medical Association)

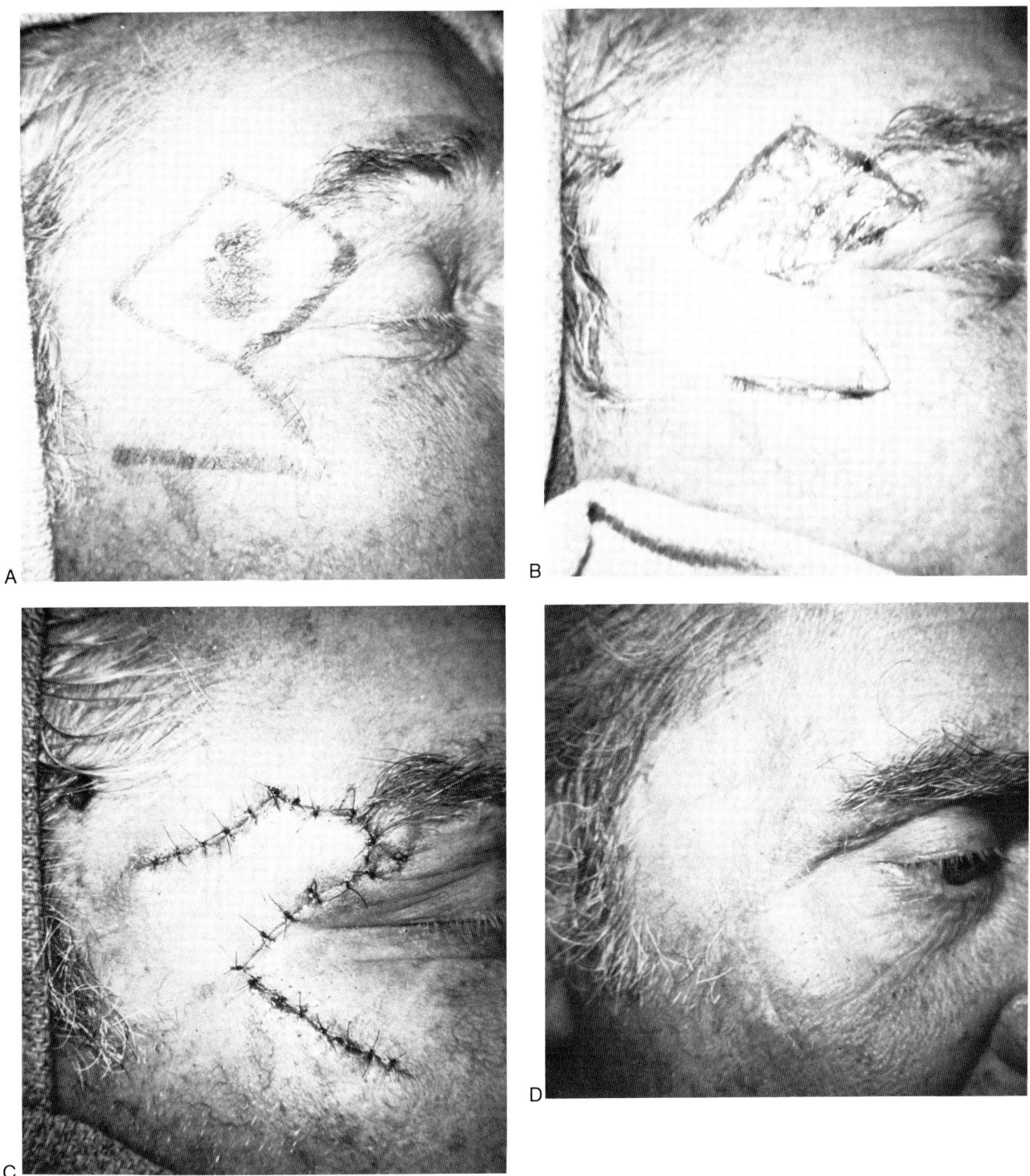

Figure 34. A, Lentigo maligna melanoma of temple; modified rhombic flap outlined (Dufourmentel). B, Tumor excised, flap elevated. C, Flap rotated into place, donor site closed. D, Final result, 4 months postoperative.

6 Bilobed Flaps

The report by Esser[1] in 1918 is believed to be the first description of a bilobed flap. He described two lobes of equal size and form. Zimmany's report[2] in 1953 described the flap in greater detail and is credited with popularizing this flap and an interest in the literature. He described a flap consisting of two lobes situated at right angles to each other on a common pedicle. He thought that a 90° angle between the two flaps was ideal, but that the angle could vary between the two lobes by as much as 45° to 80°. It should be noted that the greater the angle between the two lobes, the larger the resulting standing cutaneous cone at the point of rotation of the flap. Bilobed flaps allow one to utilize the lax tissue along the axis of both lobes of the flaps. The secondary lobe can be smaller than the primary lobe. Closure of the primary donor area is facilitated by advancing the margins of the defect of the primary lobe. The tertiary defect created by the elevation of the second lobe is closed primarily.

When using this flap, the primary lobe is planned to be the same size as the defect and the secondary lobe to be approximately half the size of the primary lobe (Figures 35, 36). Dean and colleagues[3] have stated, "The advantage of a bilobed flap is that it enables transfer of like tissue of optimal thickness and color match with minimal distortion." This advantage must be weighed against the realization that essentially two flaps are being based on one vascular pedicle and therefore the blood supply may not be as good as in a flap with a single lobe. McGregor[4] has pointed out that the approximately oval shape of each lobe of the flap can produce a degree of "pincushion effect" as an end result and that the smaller the flaps, the more likely it is to produce this "pincushioning" effect (Figure 37).

On occasion this flap is useful in the superior nasal area using glabellar skin for the donor site (Figure 38). When used in this way it creates another type of glabellar flap in addition to those already described in Chapter 4. The author does not often use bilobed flaps and tends to agree with McGregor's statement that, "all in all it has a very limited role, and is certainly not a method for the inexperienced surgeon."[4]

REFERENCES

1. Esser JFS: Gestielte lokale nasenplastik mit zweizipfligen lappen dechund des setlunderen defektes vomersten sipteldurchden zweiten. Dtsch 2 chir 143:385, 1918
2. Zimmany A: The nasolabial bilobed flap. Plast Reconstr Surg 11:424, 1952
3. Dean K, Kellerher J, Sullivan H, Baibah G: Bilobed flaps. In Grabb WC, Meyers MB (eds): Skin Flaps. Boston: Little Brown & Co, 1975
4. McGregor IA: Local skin flaps in facial reconstruction. Otolaryngol Clin North Am, 15:95–97, 1982

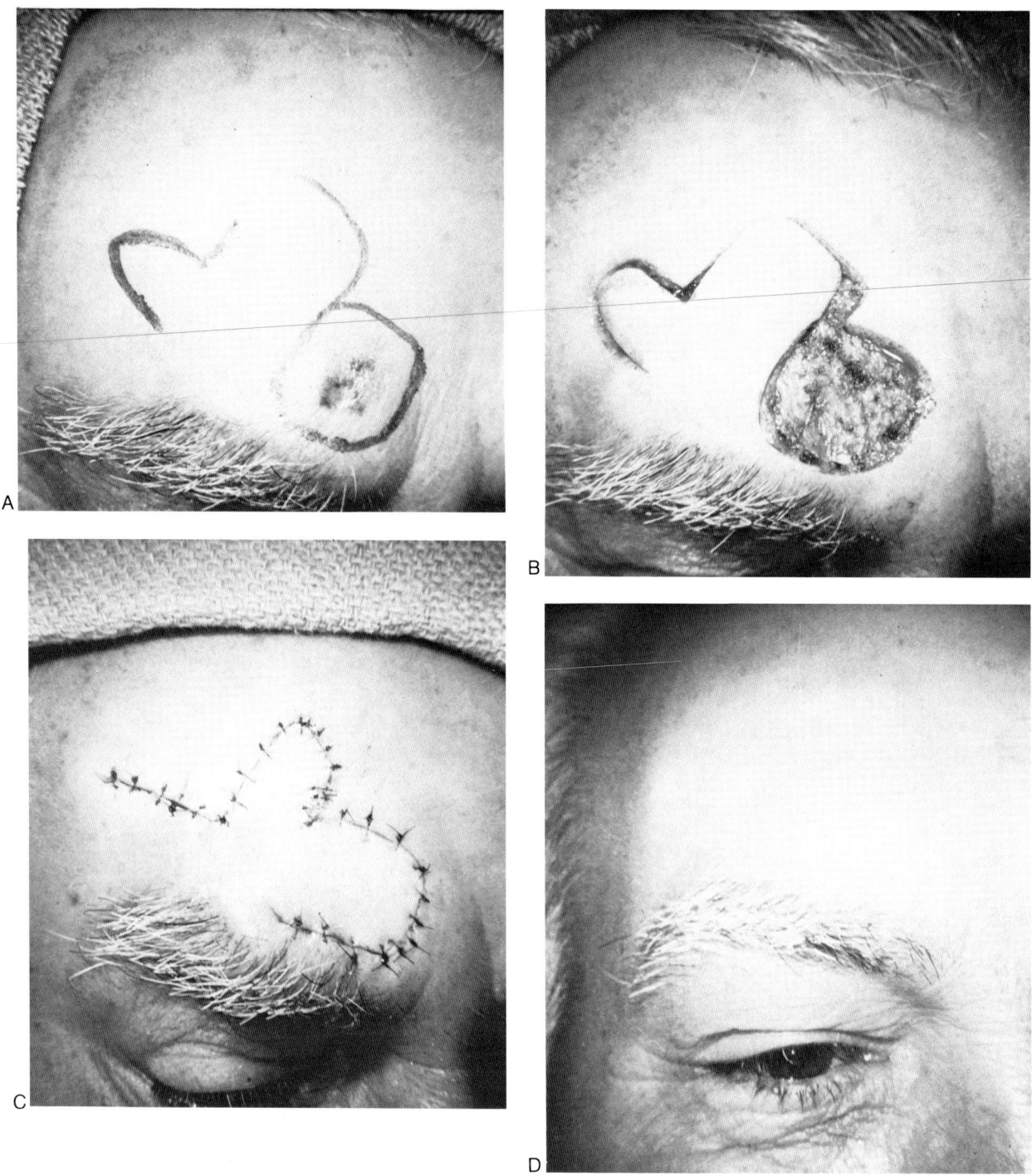

Figure 35. A, Excision of lentigo maligna marked, bilobed flap outlined. Note primary lobe same size as proposed defect, secondary lobe one-half size of primary lobe. B, Tumor excised, flap elevated. C, Flap rotated into place, donor defects closed. D, Final result, one year postoperative.

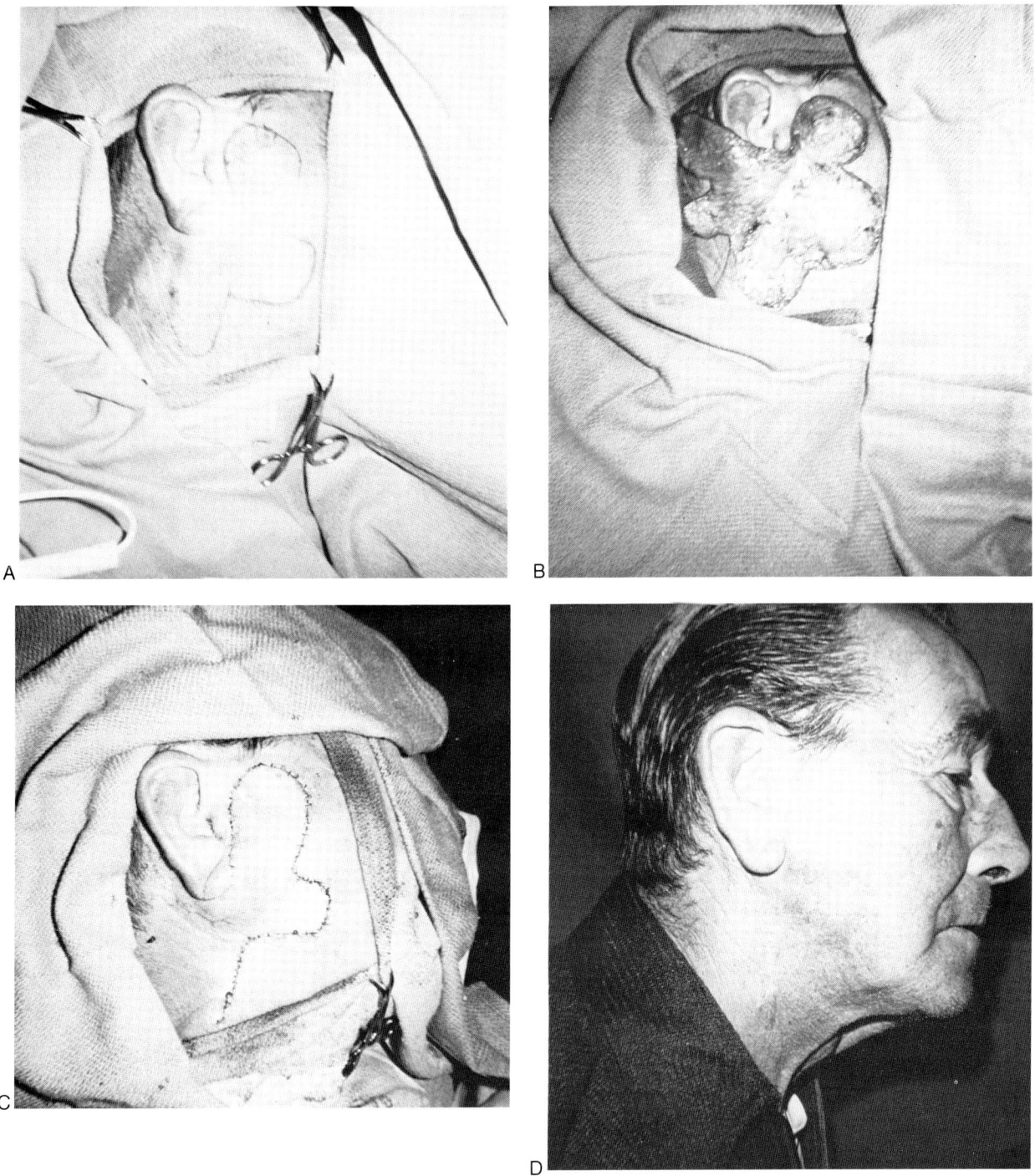

Figure 36. A, Excision of recurrent basal cell carcinoma outlined; superiorly-based bilobed flap designed. B, Tumor excised, flap elevated. C, Flap rotated into place, final closure. D, Result, one year postoperative.

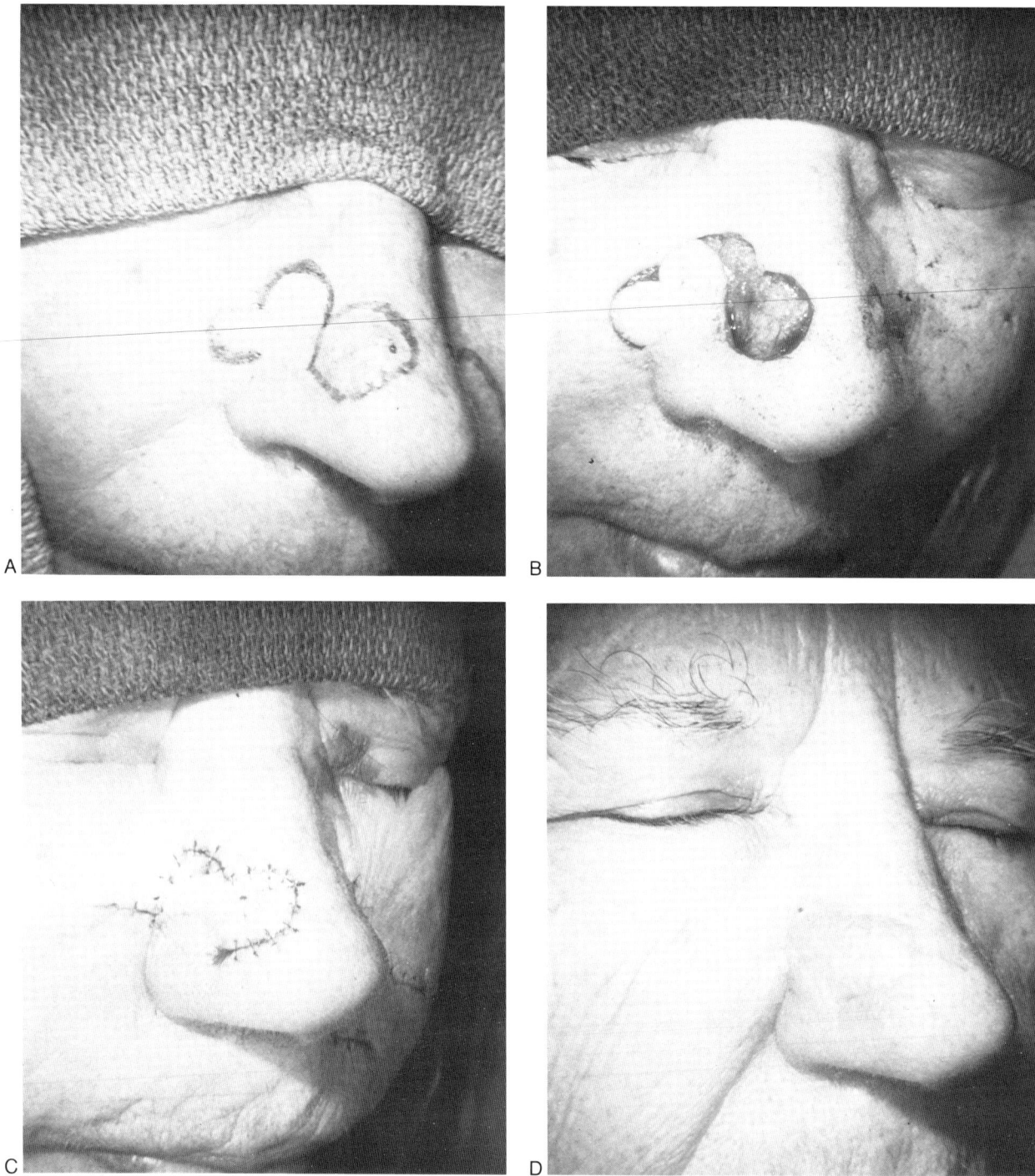

Figure 37. A, Excision basal cell carcinoma outlined; bilobed flap designed. B, Tumor excised, flap elevated. C, Flap rotated into place, donor site closed. D, Final result, one month postoperative. Note "pincushion" effect.

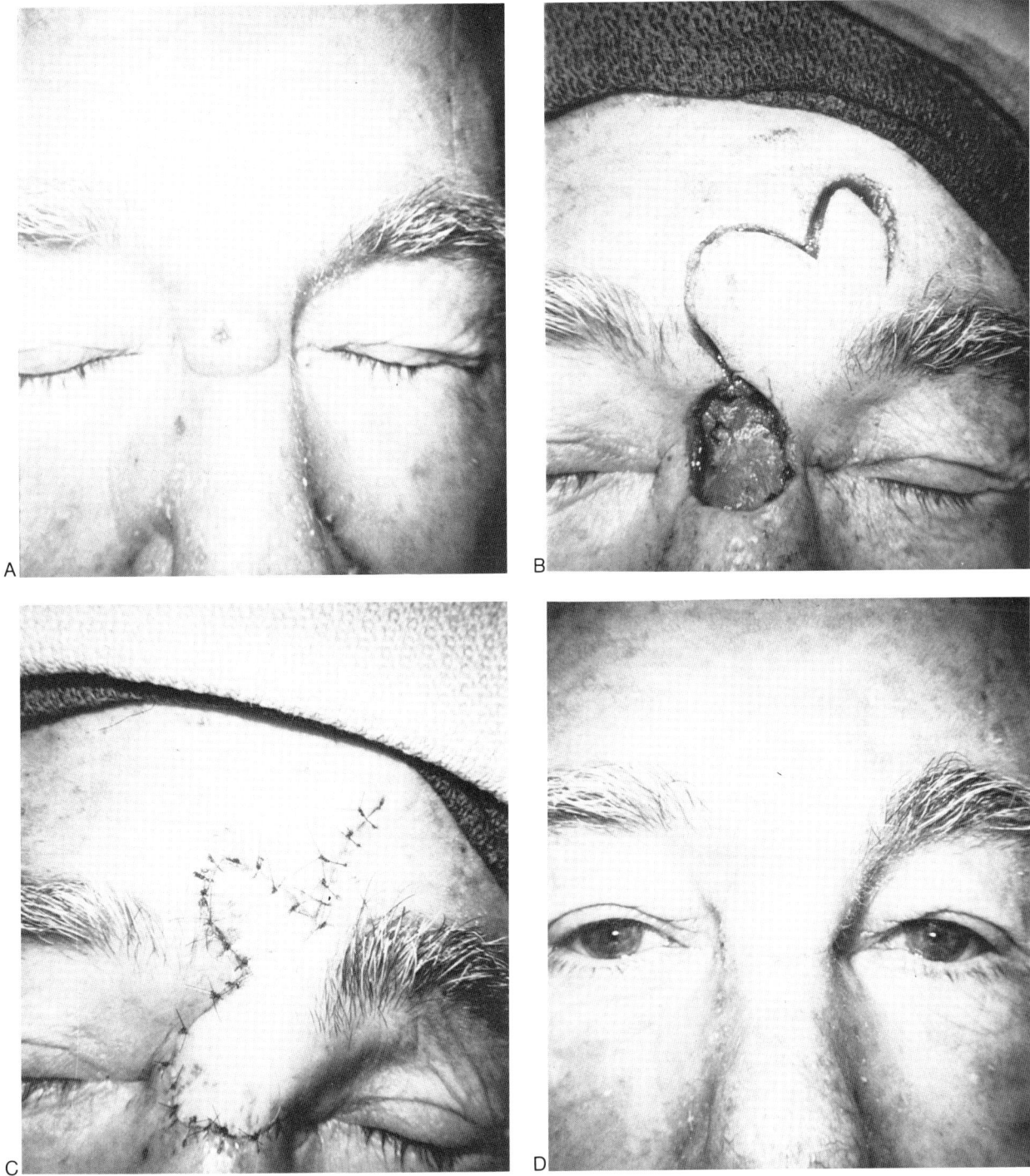

Figure 38. A, A giant keratoacanthoma of superior nasal dorsum. B, Tumor excised, bilobed glabellar flap elevated. C, Flap rotated into place, donor sites closed. D, Final result, two months postoperative.

7 Lip Flaps

The upper and lower lips are dynamic facial structures which are joined together by the oral commissures to form a major functional and aesthetic unit of the face. Unlike the nose, which is a relatively fixed facial landmark, the lips are frequently in motion with deglutition, speech, and facial expressions. Reconstruction of major lip defects creates a significant challenge to the facial surgeon in his effort to restore form and function. Further, the upper lip, with its philtrum and cupid's bow, presents a considerably more complex anatomical unit to reconstruct than the lower lip. In discussing reconstruction of the lips, it must be remembered that there are three basic layers: a middle muscular layer, an inner mucosal layer, and an outer skin layer. The latter two are joined on the outside edge of the lip at the vermilion border. The orbicularis oris muscle is a circular muscle extending around the entire circumference of the lips. It purses the lips and functions for closure in deglutition and speech. Attaching to this muscle and the skin are the various intrinsic and extrinsic muscles of the face. Their main action is in facial expression. A functioning oral commissure is vitally important in the control of salivary secretions and ingested food, making immediate reconstruction of major lip defects imperative. While an occasional skin defect of the lip may be reconstructed with a skin graft, almost all major and even many minor lip reconstructions require skin flaps. Surgical procedures to reconstruct the lips may be divided into the following categories:[1]

1. Those that use remaining lip tissue
2. Those that borrow tissue from the opposite lip
3. Those that use adjacent tissue
4. Those that use distant flaps.

Chapter 2 included the fact that an inferiorly based nasolabial flap is an excellent method to reconstruct upper lip defects involving skin and muscle only, and this type of reconstruction was illustrated in Figure 13. In Chapter 3 it was noted that cheek flaps can be used to reconstruct upper lip defects in addition to nasal defects, and this was illustrated in Figure 21. The author has even had occasion to employ a combination full thickness nasolabial and cheek flap to reconstruct a severe lower lip contracture (Figure 39). Generally, this chapter will deal with defects involving the full thickness of the lip with skin, muscle, and mucosal loss. The reconstructive modality employed will depend to a great extent on the amount of lip tissue that is missing and the location of the defect.

DEFECTS LESS THAN ONE-HALF OF THE LIP

Defects measuring less than one-half of the lip width can usually be closed with advancement of the remaining lip tissues and primary plastic repair. For a small lesion of the lip, a V-shaped excision can be planned. If the defect is going to be larger, a wedge excision with pentagonal shape should be planned and can be closed without notching, which might occur if the V-excision used is too large. If the excision appears wide, occasionally a W-plasty can be planned at the inferior aspect of the wedge to decrease the vertical length of the resulting scar. Baker and Krause[2] have cautioned that "every attempt should be made not to extend the excision beyond the mental crease, since to do so creates an unsightly pointed chin." Primary plastic closure of a lip defect must be performed in a precise manner. A muscular closure is carried out in two layers. The vermilion border is carefully approximated at the white line. Following this, mucosal and skin closure is effected. With careful closure of these primary repairs, excellent results can be expected (Figure 40). The primary closure of significant defects in the upper lip can often be facilitated by the bilateral excision of a crescentric shaped piece of cheek skin in the perialar region (Figure 41).[3] This maneuver allows advancement of the remaining lip segments while avoiding distortion of the nose and decreases the amount of tension on the wound after the closure has been carried out.

Defects of the vermilion border of the lip are often created by the excision of leukoplakia or dysplastic mucous membrane. These defects are reconstructed with mucosal advancement flaps.

Quite often when a skin cancer is removed from the lower lip, a vermilionectomy is also required. The technique for this procedure is illustrated in Figure 42. The patient in Figure 40 also had a vermilionectomy in addition to a wedge excision of the lower lip with primary enclosure.

DEFECTS GREATER THAN ONE-HALF OF THE LIP

When lip defects involve more than one-half and even the full width of the lip, augmentation is required from adjacent or regional tissues. This augmentation can be provided by a full thickness pedicle flap from either the opposite lip (lip-switch flap) or the adjacent cheeks using advancement flaps. These types of reconstructions provide static flaps that have been denervated. In recent years the Karapandzic flap[4] has become a very popular method of reconstructing moderate to large size lip defects. The Karapandzic principle involves the movement of adjacent lip flaps in to fill the defect. These flaps have the unique advantage of having their innervation and a large portion of their blood supply preserved and therefore can often provide a more dynamic and functional result than the older static flaps. Selection of flap type must be individualized. Principles of these various types of approaches to lip reconstruction will be discussed and illustrated.

Abbé-Estlander Flaps

The Abbé flap[5] was designed to close medially located defects of the lip. This is a flap consisting of the full thickness of the lip tissue including skin, muscle, and mucous membrane from the opposite lip pedicled on the vermilion border and containing the labial artery for its blood supply (Figure 43). The Abbé flap is designed to be approximately one-half the size of the opposite lip defect to be reconstructed, thereby having both lips share equally in the decrease of lip width. In three weeks or less, the flap can safely be divided and the vermilion borders can be reapproximated.

The Estlander flap[6] (Figure 44) was designed for closure of a lip defect near the commissure of the mouth. As with the Abbé flap, the width of the flap is approximately one-half that of the defect, so that the lips are reduced proportionately. Great care should be taken to protect the labial artery that provides the blood supply to the flap. As mentioned, with primary closure, meticulous attention should be used to approximate the vermilion border of the flap as part of the three layer closure in order to prevent notching. Many variations of the Abbé and Estlander flaps have been devised including combining the Abbé flap with advancement cheek flaps for large defects.[7]

Adjacent Cheek Flaps

The classic approach to the reconstruction of large defects of the middle of the lower lip has been the Bernard[8] operation. The modification of this operation by Ginestet[9] is the most efficacious in using this technique for large defects (Figure 45). The principles of this operation involve the advancement of cheek flaps, which are incised horizontally in a posterior direction at the level of the lateral commissures, out past the nasolabial folds as far as is necessary to advance the two sides together. To allow this advancement, triangles of skin, subcutaneous tissue, and some muscle are removed from the cheek, with their medial borders located along the nasolabial folds and their lateral borders on the cheek, causing the closure to be hidden in the nasolabial folds. The mucosa on the back of these triangles is preserved, pedicled inferiorly, and folded over the new flap to create the mucous membrane portion of the lip and the vermilion border. The lower mucosal incision is made along the gingivo-buccal sulcus bilaterally back to the last molar tooth. A triangle of tissue is removed on both sides of the defect, below and lateral to it, to allow the flaps to advance medially after they are undermined widely at a depth just superficial to the periosteum of the bone of the mandible. This elevation has to be carried quite far posteriorly on occasion to allow a closure without undue tension. This method has the added advantage of support of the newly created lower lip by the sling-like effect of the bilateral flaps. For the same reason, there exists the possibility of a pouting appearance of the relatively longer upper lip. An additional disadvantage is the denervation of the orbicularis oris muscle, which makes the newly created lip unit a more static anatomical structure. While certainly not perfect, this operation has stood the test of time and is still an excellent method for lower lip reconstruction.

Innervated Musculocutaneous Lip Flaps (Karapandzic)

In 1974, Karapandzic[4] reported the use of arterialized innervated advancement lip flaps for the reconstruction of major lip defects. This new and innovative technique captured the imagination of many facial surgeons who have been employing it with increasing enthusiasm. The objective of the operation is to separate two flaps of skin and orbicularis muscle, which are left attached to the mucous membrane and to their feeding arterioles and nerves. These two flaps are advanced together to create the newly reconstructed lip (Figure 46). The skin incisions are planned to extend horizontally and laterally from the base of the newly created defect, and the flaps are made as wide as the height of the defect. Laterally the incisions are carried into the nasolabial folds. After the defect has been created, the incisions for the flaps are made through the skin and subcutaneous tissue. The intrinsic and extrinsic muscles are separated below the incision with blunt dissection to preserve the nerves and vessels that approach the lip perpendicularly. As many of the major small nerves and vessels as possible are preserved. Necessarily, a few small nerves and vessels are probably sacrificed.

The muscles are completely separated at the incision site down to the mucous membrane of the buccal mucosa, which is carefully preserved and not incised. Because the mucous membrane is quite mobile it is not necessary to incise it, and preservation of this structure enhances the blood supply of the flap. The flaps are advanced medially and sutured into place with a three layered closure, as with any full thickness lip defect. Both flaps must be incised and mobilized to prevent asymmetry of the mouth. When the dissection is complete, the ends should meet quite easily without tension. Following the lip reconstruction, the donor defect is closed directly by the halving technique and the removal of the standing cone laterally, if necessary. The major advantage of this operation is the reconstruction of a lip with adjacent lip tissue, which is vascularized and innervated and can function with normal sphincter control of a mouth with a smaller circumference. The main disadvantage seems to be the creation of microstomia when very large defects are reconstructed using this principle. The operation can be used to correct large defects of the lower lip as illustrated in Figures 46 and 47, and can also be used to reconstruct large defects of the upper lip, as in Figure 48.

When the defect involves an entire lip and a portion or portions of the mandible or maxilla, distant flaps and more recently free flaps are required for the reconstruction. These types of reconstructions are beyond the scope of this monograph on local and regional flaps.

REFERENCES

1. Kazanjian VH, Converse JM: The Surgical Treatment of Facial Injuries, 2nd ed. Baltimore. Williams & Wilkins, 1959
2. Baker SR, Krause CJ: Pedicle flaps in reconstruction of the lip. Facial Plast Surg 1:61–68, 1983
3. Webster JP: Crescentric peri-alar cheek excision for upper lip flap advancement with a short history of upper lip repair. Plast Reconstr Surg 16:434, 1955
4. Karapandzic M: Reconstruction of lip defects by local arterial flaps. Nr J Plast Sur 27:93, 1974
5. Abbé R: A new plastic operation for the relief of deformity due to double hairlip. Med Rec 53:477, 1898
6. Estlander JA: Eine methode aud der einen lippe substanzverluste der anderen zu erstegen. Arch Klin Chir 14:622, 1872
7. Converse JA(ed.): Reconstructive Plastic Surgery, 2nd ed. Philadelphia London Toronto: W B Saunders, 1977
8. Bernard C: Cancer de la levre inferieure opere par un procede nouveau. Bull Soc Chir 3:357, 1853
9. Ginestet G: Reconstruction de toute la levre inferieure par les lambeaux naso-geniens totaux. Revue d'Odontologie et Stomatologie 8:28, 1946

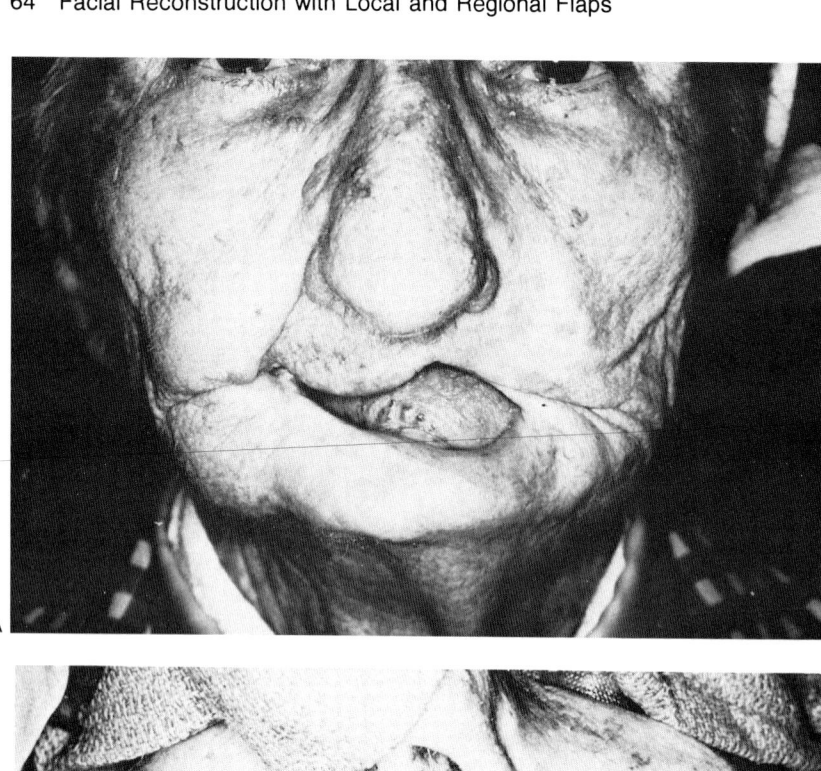
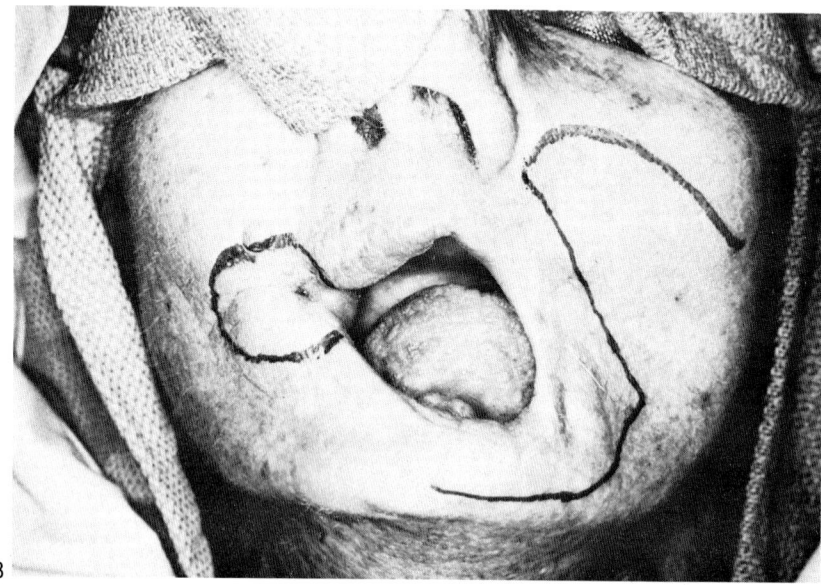
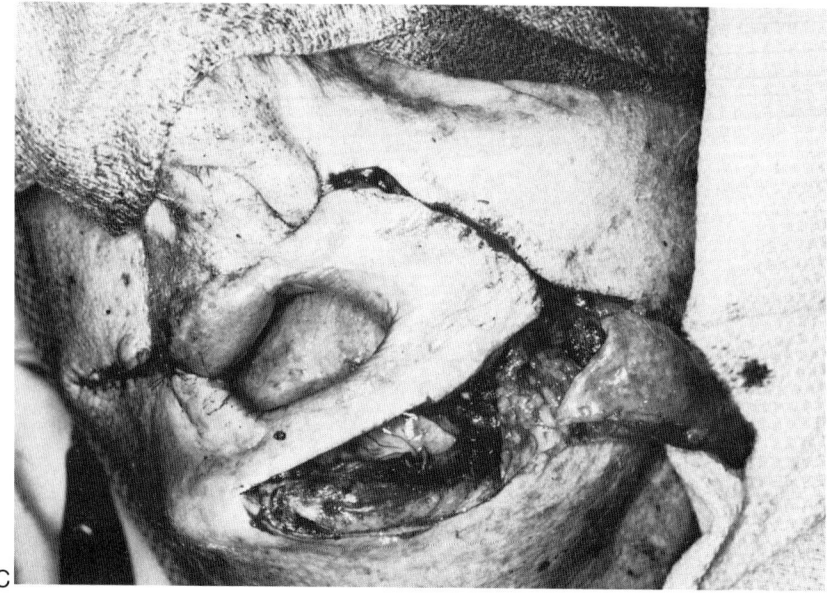

Figure 39. A, Severe left lower lip contracture secondary to previous surgery by another physician. B, Full thickness nasolabial-cheek flap outlined; excision of another large primary squamous cell carcinoma of the right oral commissure also outlined. C, Scar contracture released, full thickness flap elevated.

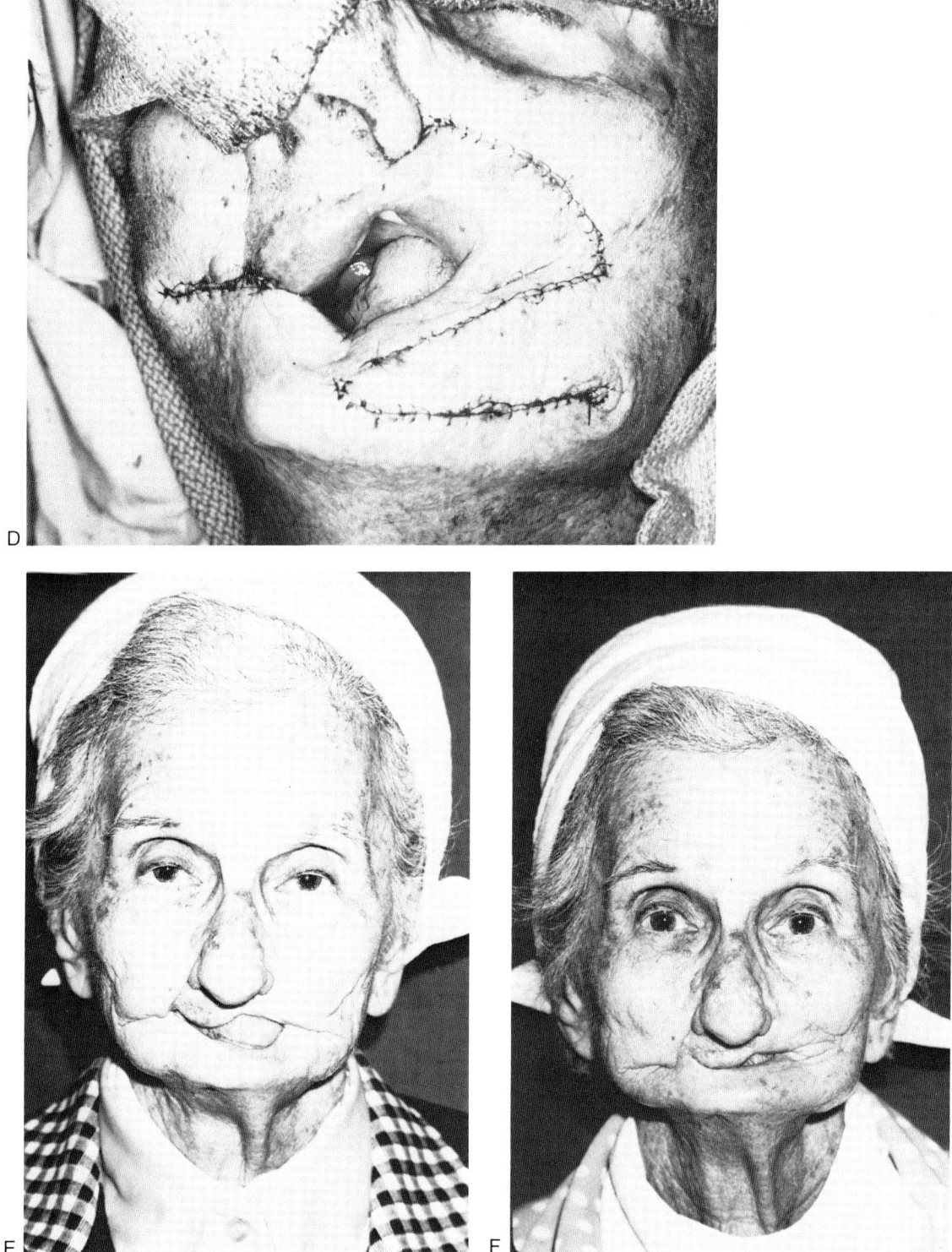

Figure 39. (cont.) D, Flap transposed. E, Full face, preoperative. F, Result, two months postoperative.

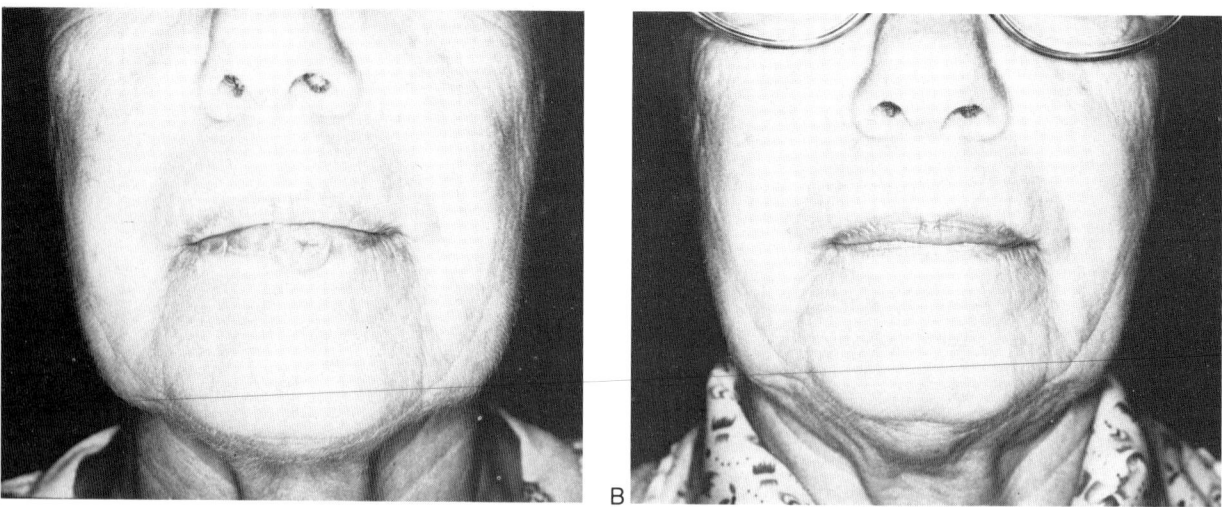

Figure 40. A, Squamous cell carcinoma of lower lip with dysplasia and carcinoma-in-situ at the adjacent vermillion border. B, Appearance following wedge excision with primary closure and vermilionectomy, three months postoperative.

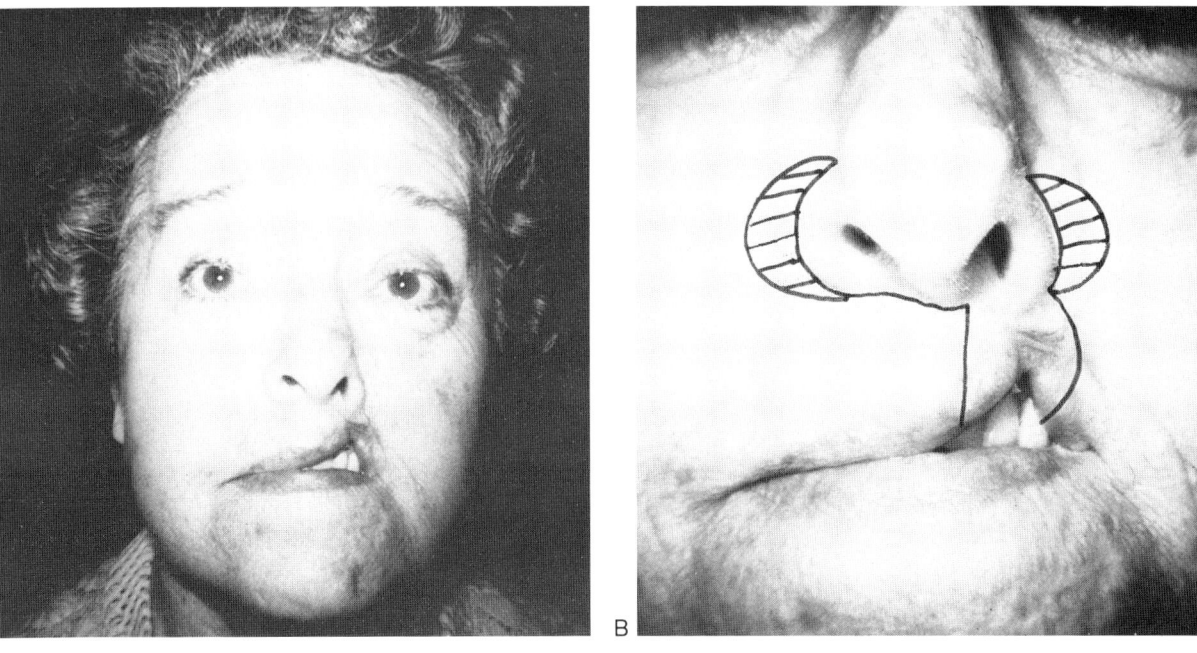
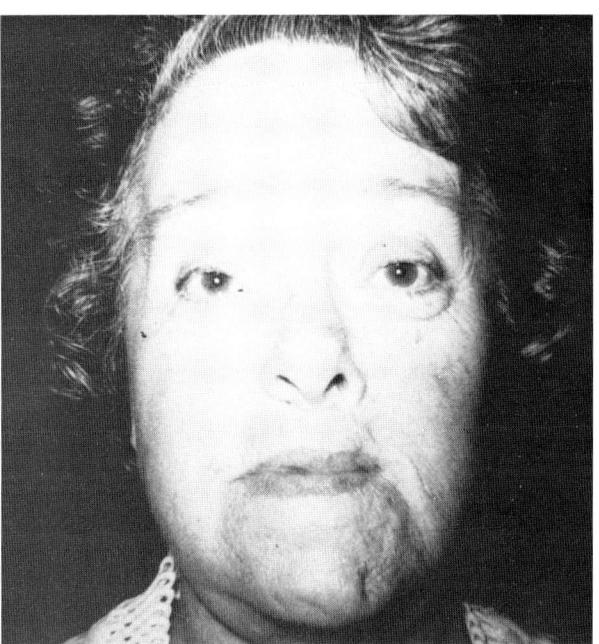

Figure 41. A, Severe contracture of upper lip secondary to extensive Mohs' surgery by another surgeon. B, Closure facilitated by bilateral excision of crescentric shaped perialar tissue blocks. C, Final appearance, six months postoperative. (Reprinted with permission from: Becker FF: Reconstruction of facial defects resulting from Mohs' chemosurgical procedures. Dermatol Surg Oncol 4:73, 1978)

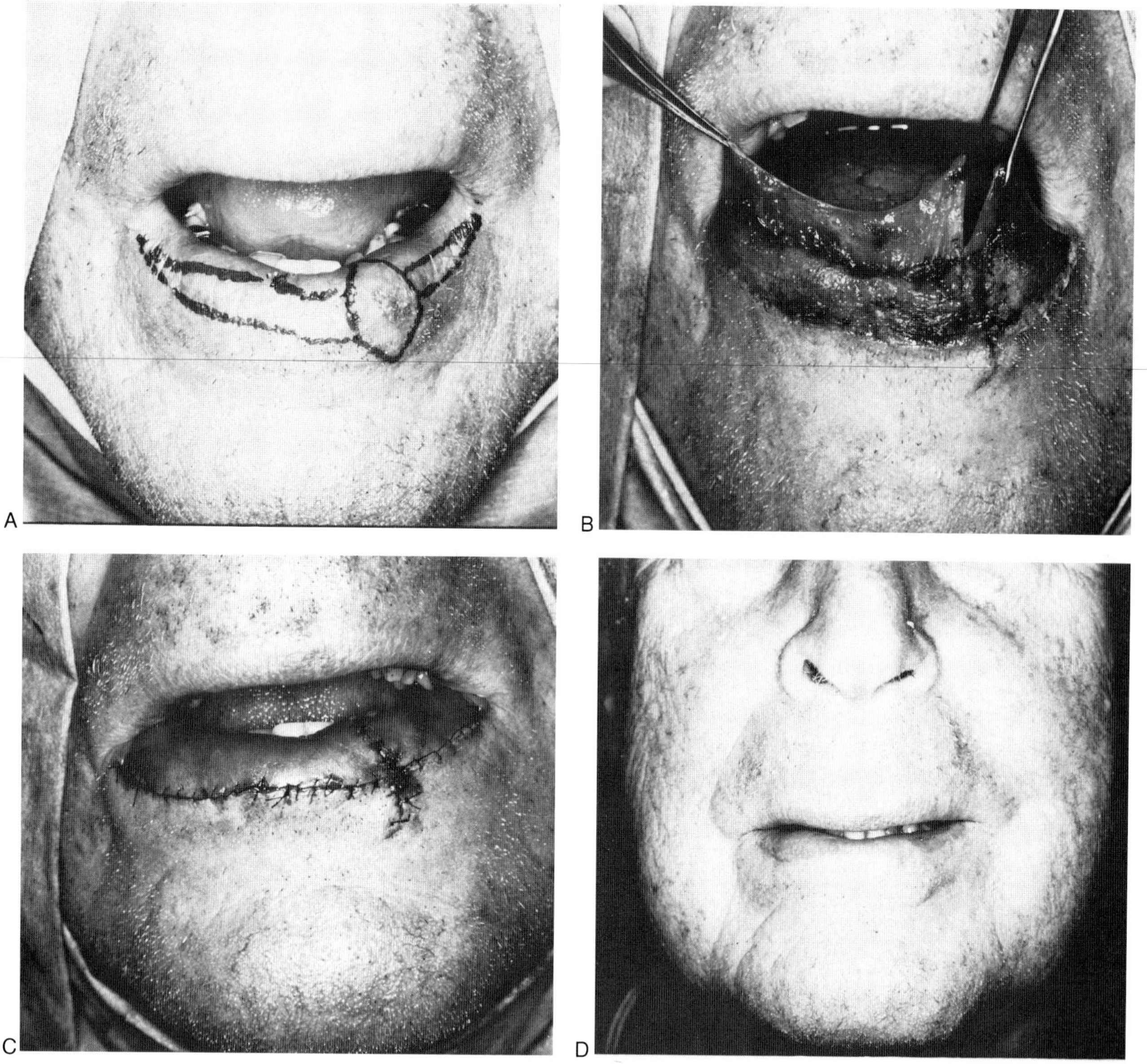

Figure 42. A, Small squamous cell carcinoma of lower lip with severe dysplasia of entire lower lip; excisions outlined. B, Tumors excised, mucosal flap elevated. C, Final closure. D, Result, six months postoperative.

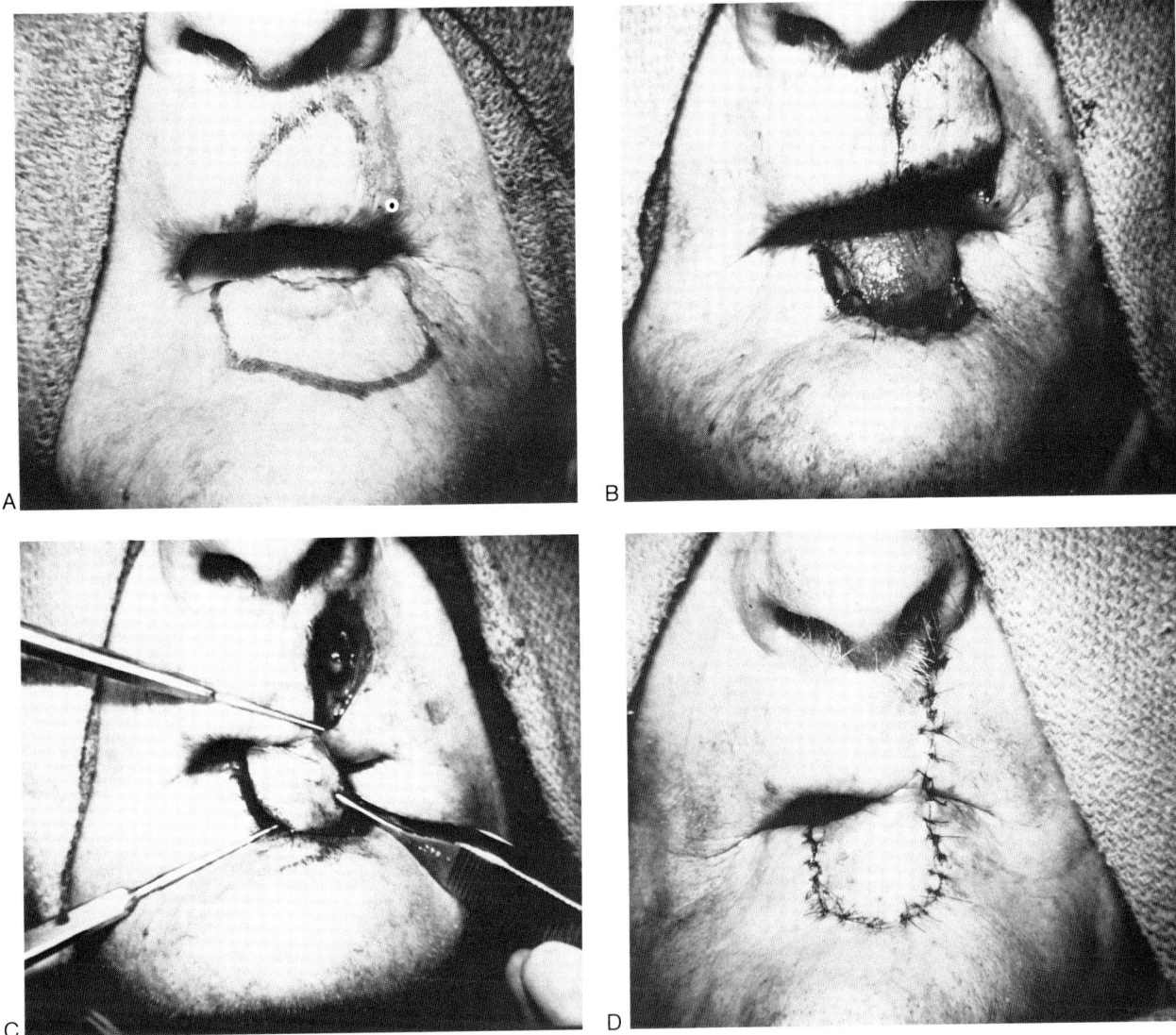

Figure 43. A, Large squamous cell carcinoma of lower lip; proposed excision marked requiring excision of more than two-thirds of lower lip; Abbé flap outlined. B, Tumor excised; flap incised through lip except at pedicle which contains labial artery. C, Flap rotated into position. D, Final closure.

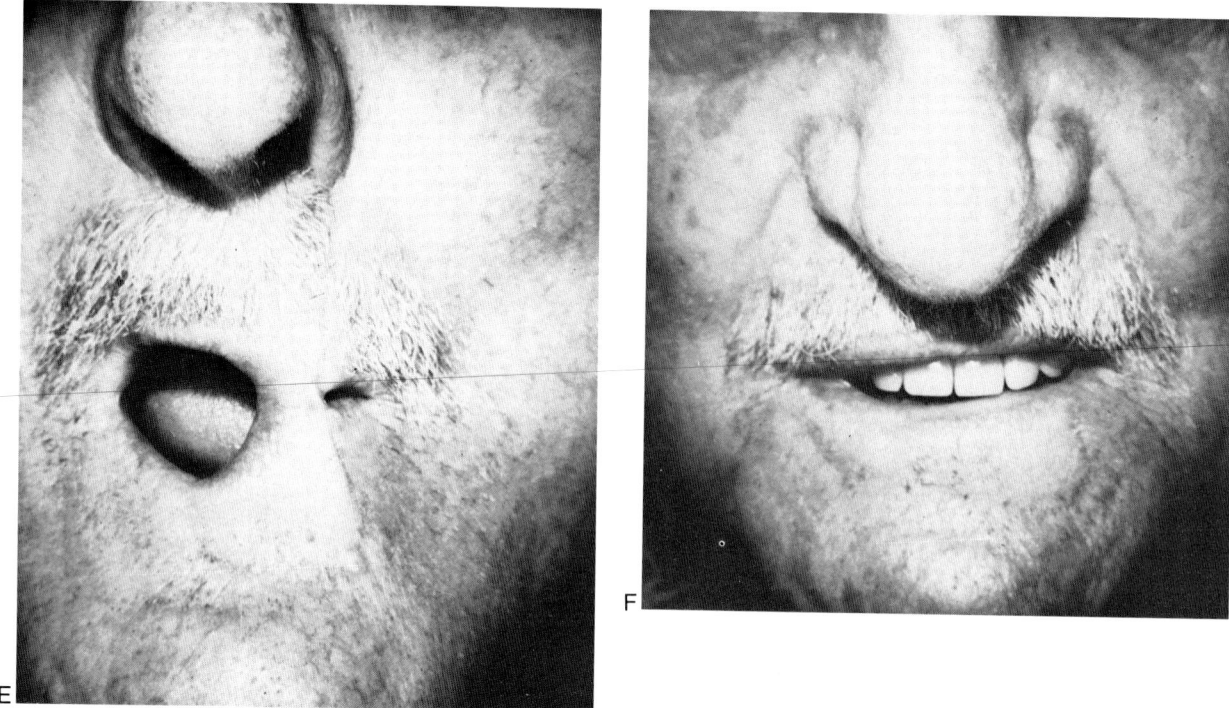

Figure 43. (cont.) E, Appearance three weeks postoperative, immediately prior to secondary releasing procedure. F, Result, four months postoperative.

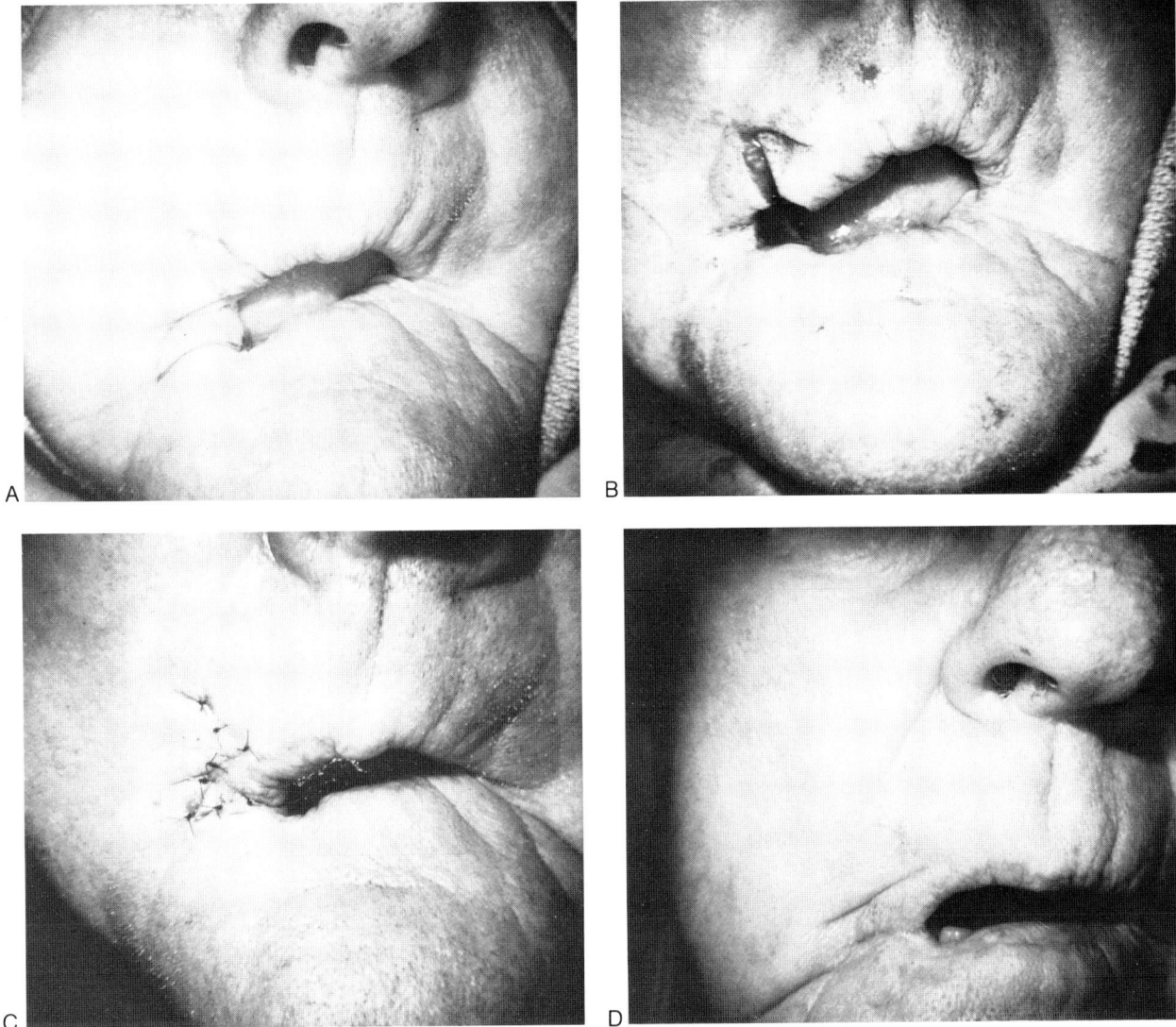

Figure 44. A, Recurrent squamous cell carcinoma of right lower lip and lateral commissure; excision and Estlander flap outlined. B, Tumor excised into buccal mucosa; flap incised with pedicle based medially on labial artery. C, Flap rotated into place, donor site closed. D, Result, two months postoperative.

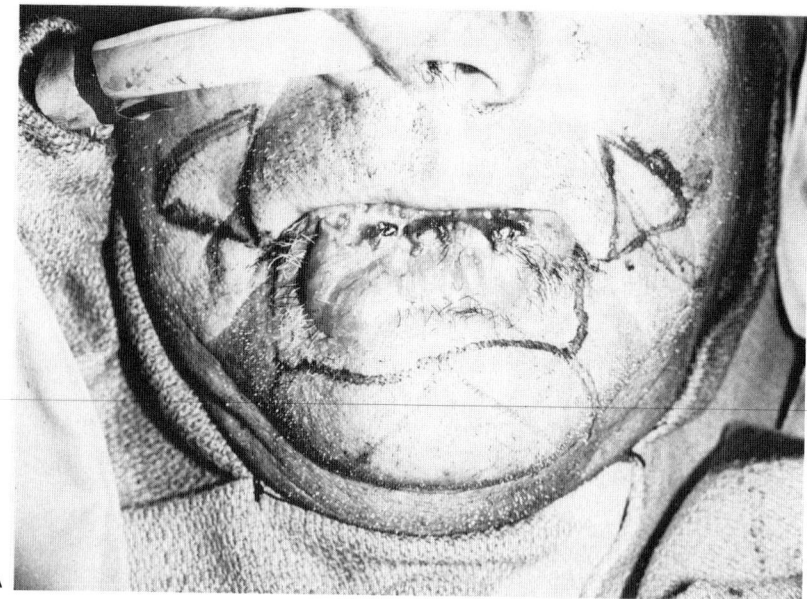
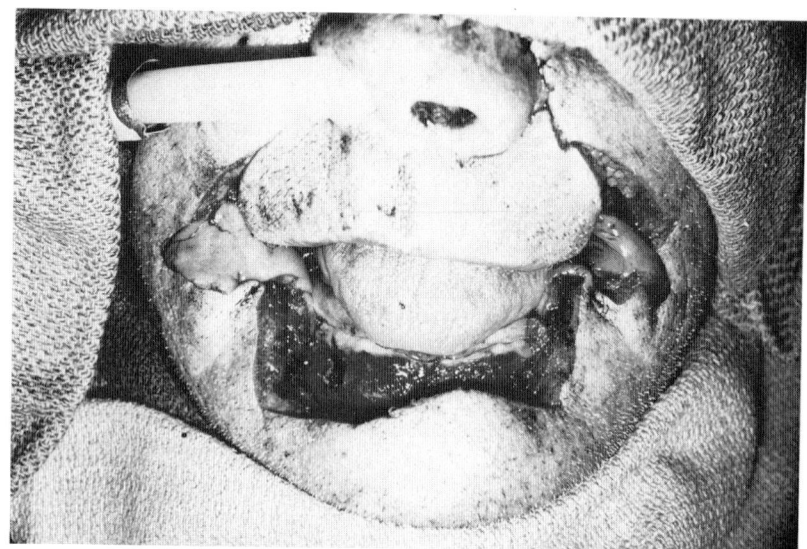
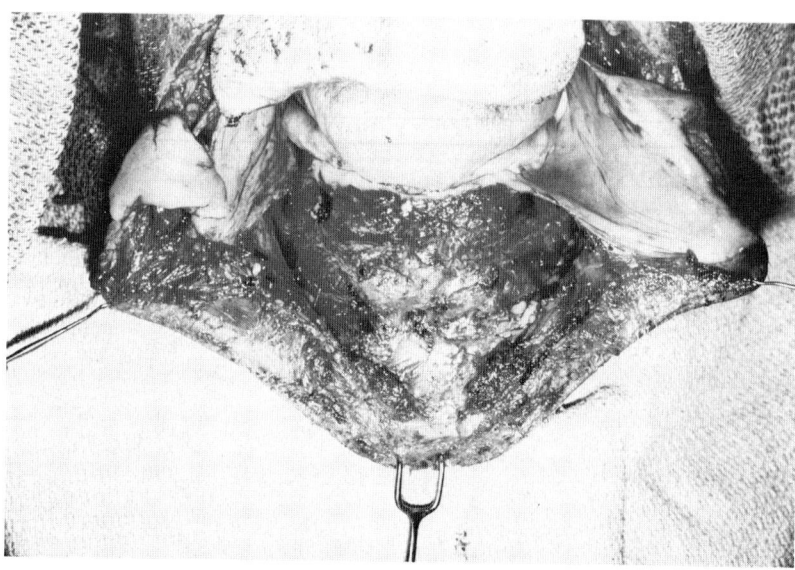

Figure 45. A, Enormous squamous cell carcinoma involving entire lower lip and adjacent tissue; Ginestet modification of Bernard chieloplasty outlined. B, Tumor excised, nasolabial wedges excised, mucosal flaps advanced forward. C, Extent of elevation.

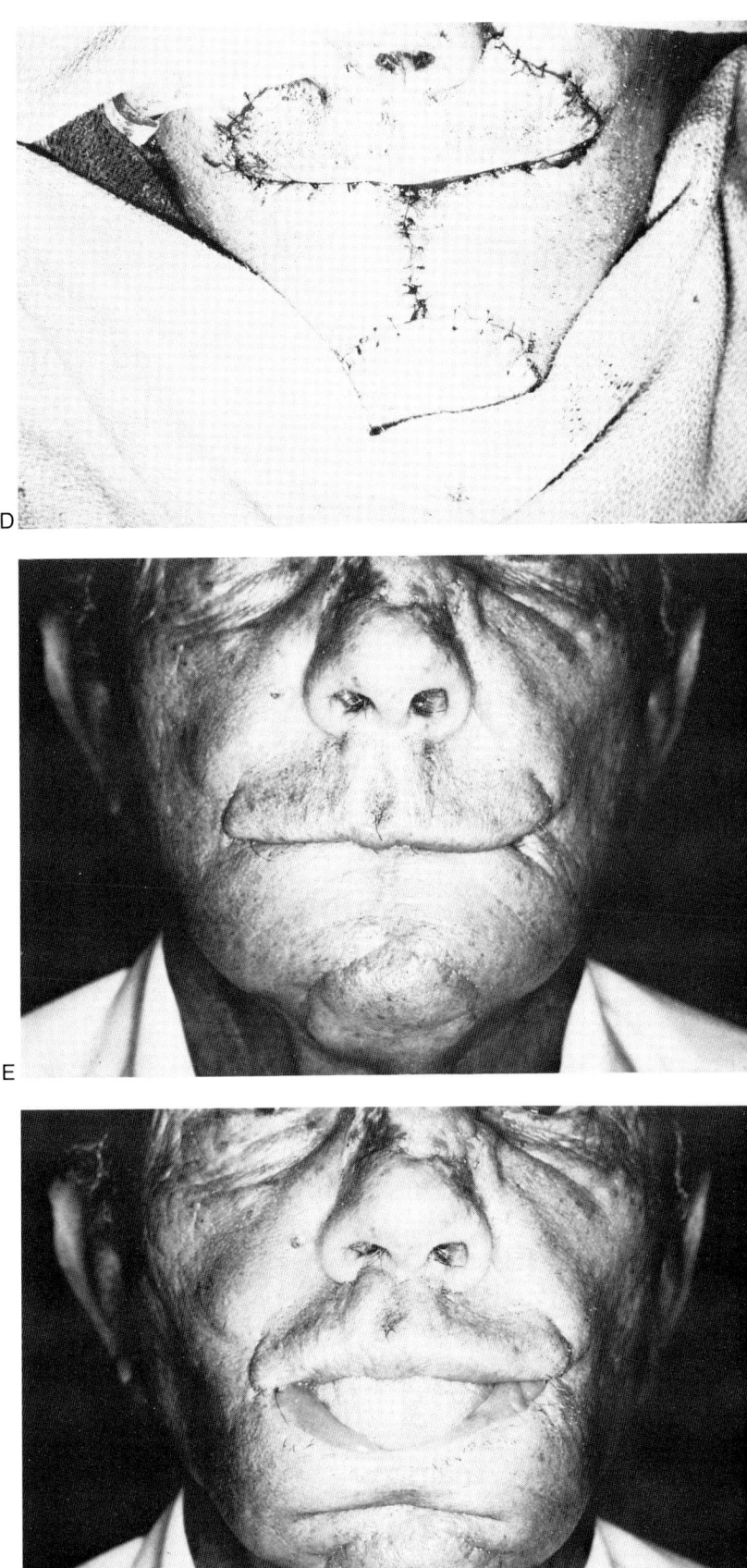

Figure 45. (cont.) D, Final closure. E, Final result, two months postoperative, in repose. F, Final result, two months postoperative, mouth open, tongue thrust forward.

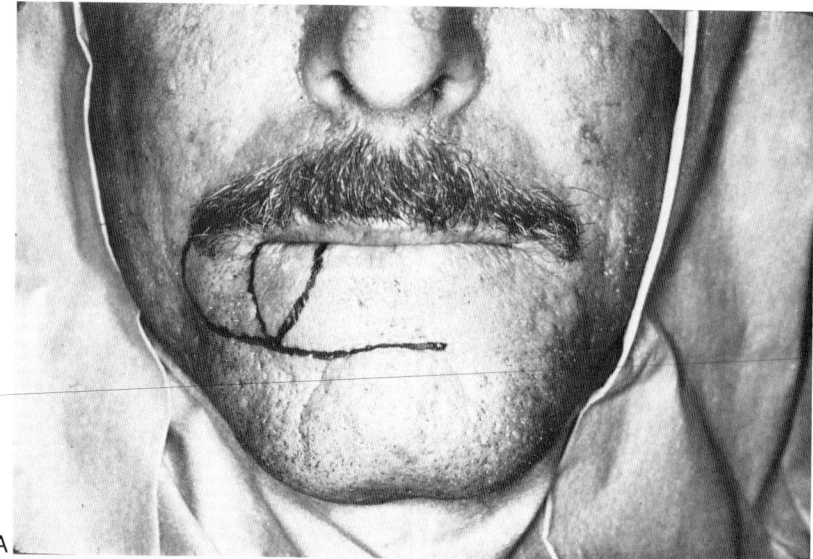
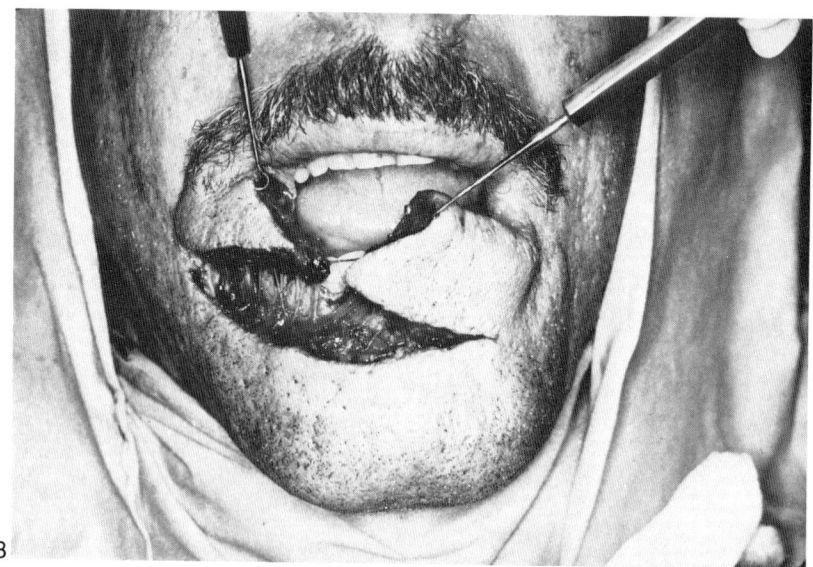
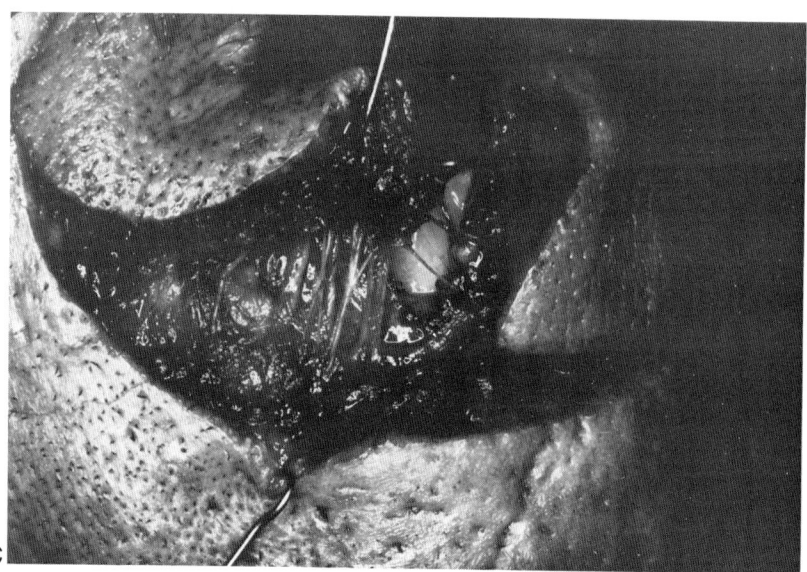

Figure 46. A, Squamous cell carcinoma right lower lip, previous wedge excision with tumor in margin two weeks prior to this procedure. Estimated combined total loss, more than half of lower lip. Karapanzic flaps, outlined. B, Tumor excised, flaps elevated with the preservation of mucous membrane. C, Right flap with neural and vascular structures preserved.

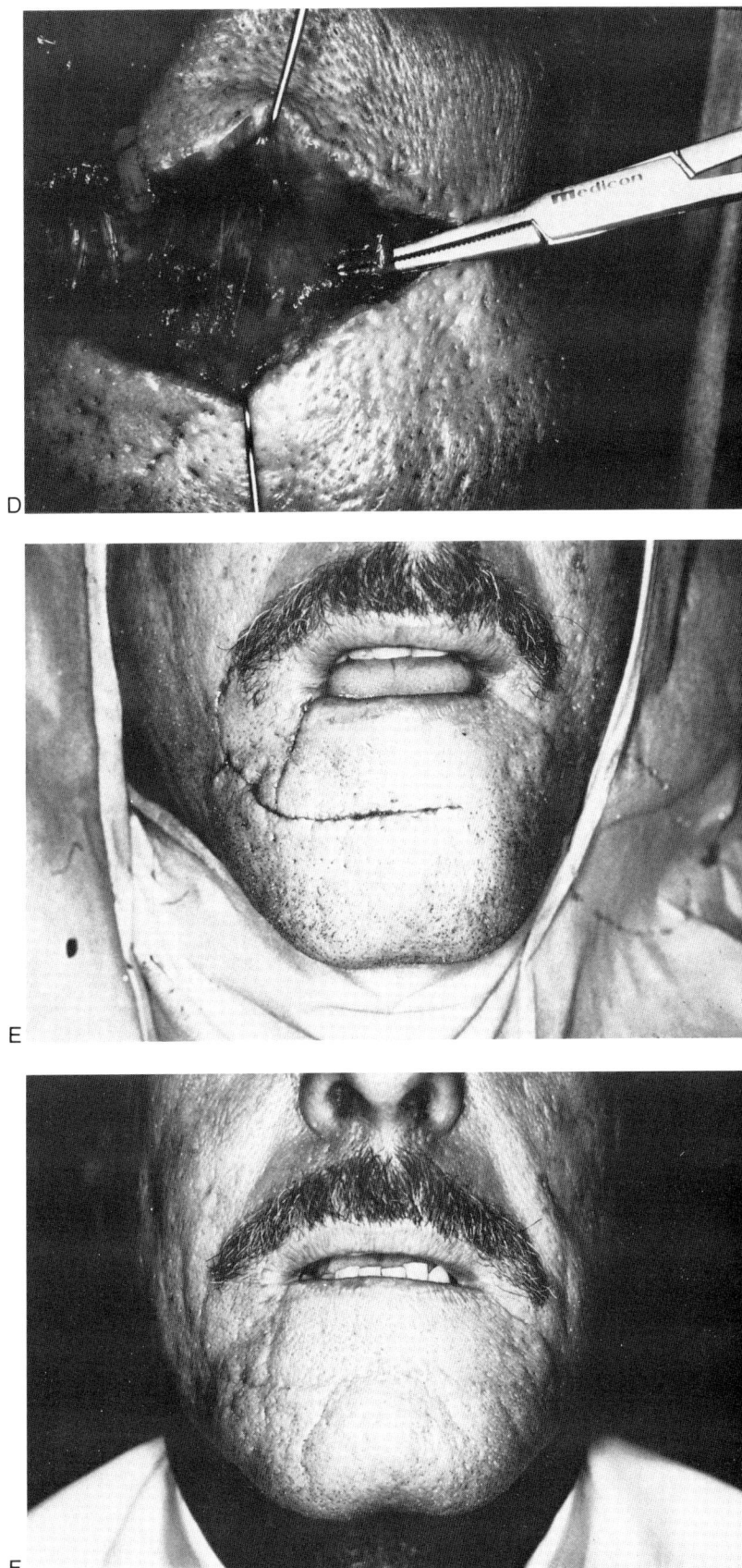

Figure 46. (cont.) D, Left flap with hemostat under artery. E, Final closure. F, Result, six months postoperative.

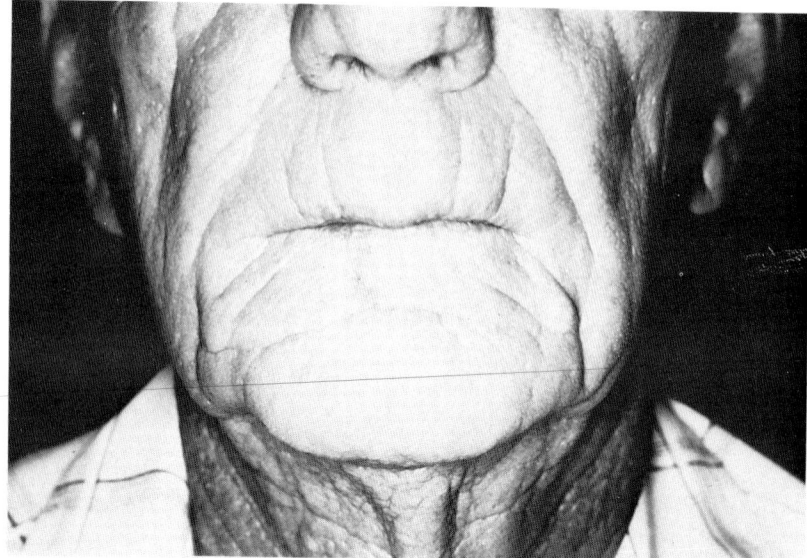

Figure 47. Postoperative six months, total reconstruction of lower lip with Karapanzic flaps.

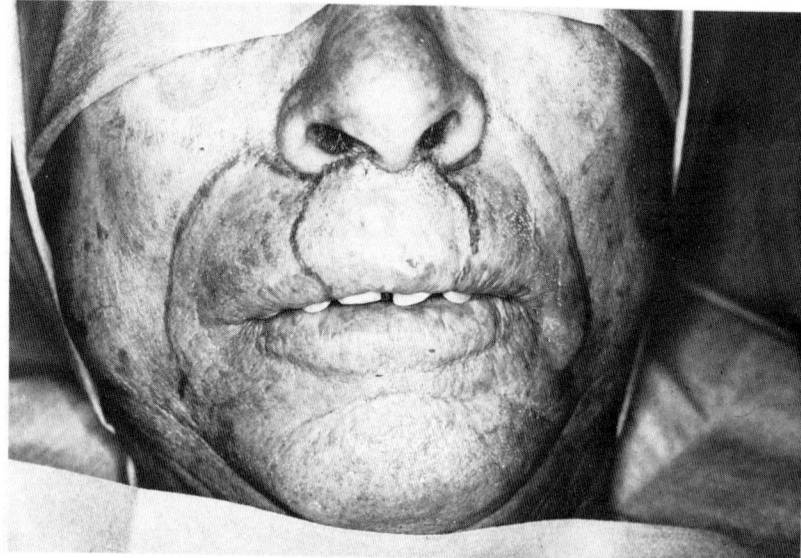

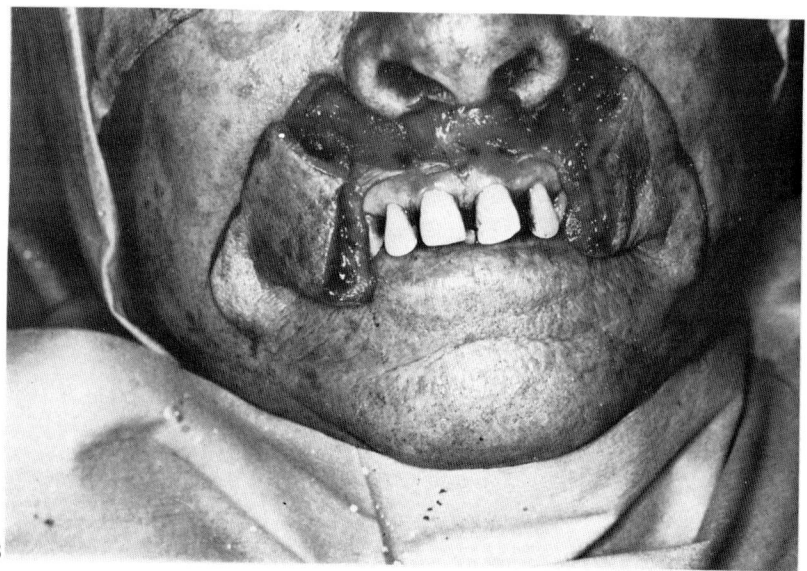

Figure 48. A, Squamous cell carcinoma through-and-through upper lip following surgical excisions and radiation therapy by other physicians; excision and Karapanzic flaps outlined. B, Tumor excised by Mohs' technique; flaps elevated.

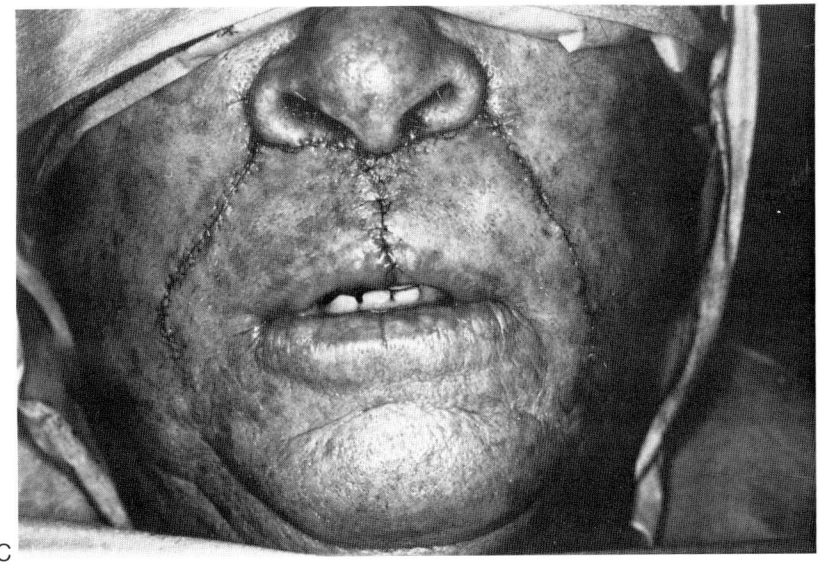

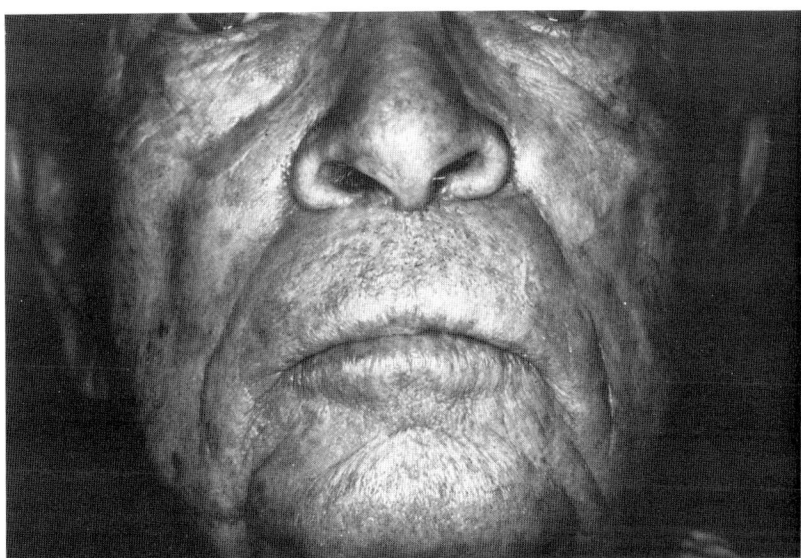

Figure 48. (cont.) C, Final closure. D, Result, one month postoperative.

8 Eyelid Reconstruction

The eyelids are delicate and anatomically intricate structures. The physiological functions of the eyelids with their specialized muscles and secretory mechanisms are quite complex. Whole books and chapters are written on the anatomy and physiology of the eyelids and these subjects are beyond the scope of this monograph. However, before embarking on any reconstructive procedure of the eyelids, the facial surgeon should have a sound knowledge of the anatomy and physiology of these structures. For purposes of this chapter, it is assumed that the reader has already developed this foundation. A few basic points on the surgical anatomy of the eyelids will be reviewed.

The eyelids are divided into an outer musculocutaneous layer containing the skin and orbicularis muscle and an inner tarsoconjunctival layer composed of tarsus and conjunctiva. These two layers are divided at the mid margin by the gray line. The upper and lower eyelids are joined by a medial and a lateral canthal tendon at the medial and lateral canthi. The anatomy of the medial canthus is more complicated than that of the lateral canthus owing to the caruncle, puncta, canaliculi and lacrimal drainage system.

The lids not only have the important function of protecting the cornea and globe, but they also constitute a vitally important and highly visible aesthetic unit of the face. Therefore, reconstruction of lost lid tissue is extremely important to protect the eye and to give the patient an acceptable appearance. Unlike the lips, many defects of the outer lining of the eyelids involving skin and muscle are appropriately reconstructed with full thickness skin grafts.

Reconstruction of the eyelids with flaps is comparable in a number of ways to the reconstruction of lips, which was discussed in the previous chapter. These types of reconstructions involve procedures with the following concepts: (1) use of remaining lid tissues, (2) borrowing tissues from the lid opposite from the defect, (3) adjacent tissue flap reconstructions, and (4) distant flap reconstructions. In full thickness eyelid reconstructions, it is imperative to provide an inner lining of mucous membrane to protect the cornea and, for large defects, some type of structural support for the loss of tarsus. In this way, eyelid reconstructions are more complex than lip reconstructions since there is very little excess tissue and the structures are considerably more delicate. The procedures must be performed with much more care because they are carried out with the cornea and globe at risk.

Reconstruction of eyelid defects can be divided into relatively superficial defects, involving only skin or skin and muscle up to the lash margin, and full thickness defects, involving both the musculocutaneous layer and the tarsoconjunctival layer. A discussion of flap reconstructions of these two types of defects will be carried out separately.

FLAP RECONSTRUCTION OF EYELID DEFECTS INVOLVING SKIN AND MUSCLE

Since there is so little excess tissue available in the eyelids, defects of the skin and muscle of any appreciable size often cannot be closed primarily. For the same reason, there is very little local lid skin to advance or transpose for a flap on the involved eyelid. Occasionally it is possible to perform an advancement eyelid flap to reconstruct a skin or skin muscle defect (Figure 49). This same type of flap may be used instead of a skin graft on occasion for skin muscle replacement in a total lower eyelid reconstruction by the Hughes technique (Figure 59), which is discussed later in this chapter. It has already been noted in Chapter 3 that laterally advanced or rotated cheek tissue can be used to reconstruct musculocutaneous defects of the eyelid. Figure 18 illustrates such a reconstruction.

Besides the adjacent cheek, the most readily available local skin for flaps to the lower eyelid is from the upper eyelid. Figure 50 represents a case in which there was tissue loss of the lower eyelid, particularly laterally, creating an ectropion. This problem was reconstructed with a laterally based upper eyelid flap. The technique not only provides the missing tissue which is of like texture and color match, but also created a sling-like effect since the base of the flap is located superiorly helping with the ectropion correction. (This procedure was also illustrated in Figure 22E–J in Chapter 3.) The reconstruction of a medial lower eyelid ectropion is made more complicated by the presence of the lacrimal drainage system and medial canthal tendon in this area. Anderson[1] in 1978 described an excellent technique for the reconstruction of medial lower eyelid ectropion utilizing a medially based upper eyelid flap (Figure 51). As part of this technique, a plication of the lower crus of the medial canthal tendon must be carried out. As with the laterally based flap, this flap provides tissue of like color and texture match and a sling-like effect that enhances the ectropion correction. Because forehead skin is much thicker and more coarse than eyelid skin, forehead flaps are not recommended for the reconstruction of eyelid defects because these flaps give a bulky and unnatural appearance to the eyelids (Figure 52). This is in direct opposition to some of the previous literature on eyelid reconstruction.

FLAP RECONSTRUCTION OF FULL THICKNESS EYELID DEFECTS

Full thickness defects of the eyelids require a reconstruction that provides replacement for both the inner, tarsoconjunctival layer and the outer, musculocutaneous layer. When the defect is small or located medially or laterally, the inner layer can occasionally be provided by advancement of the conjunctiva of the fornix to provide a mucous secreting lining (Figure 53). When the full thickness defect involves a significant portion of the central part of the lid, an inner lining providing both a mucous membrane layer and a supporting layer to replace the tarsus must be provided, as well as an outer layer to replace the skin and muscle. If the full thickness defect of the eyelid measures less than one-fourth of the lid width, a primary closure can usually be effected. If necessary, additional horizontal lid length can be provided by a lateral cantholysis in which the inferior crus of the lateral canthal tendon is severed. The technique of primary closure and lateral cantholysis is illustrated in Figure 54. This type of closure is comparable to the primary closure of a small to moderate sized full thickness lower lip defect, but is more intricate. The tarsal layer is closed with a long-acting absorbable suture. A good tarsal closure should approximate the conjunctiva. One must be careful not to bury any knots in a way that would touch the cornea. After the tarsal layer has been closed, three sutures are placed through the lid margin at the inner margin (white line), the gray line and the lash line. The inner two sutures are brought outward and their ends are tied over the outermost suture at the lash line to prevent the sutures from irritating the cornea. The skin is then closed appropriately.

Most of the remaining portion of this chapter will deal with the two basic methods of reconstructing large full thickness defects of the lower eyelids, which have been found to be the most useful in these deformities. The Hughes[2] procedure involves the transfer of a tarsoconjunctival flap from the upper eyelid to reconstruct an inner lining for the lower eyelid defect, and an outer lining is provided by either a full thickness skin graft or an inferiorly based advancement flap from the remaining eyelid. The other approach to total lower eyelid reconstruction is that of Mustardé[3] which involves a chondromucosal composite graft from the nasal septum for inner lining and an inferiorly based rotation cheek flap for outer lining.

Two schools of thought have developed regarding the best technique of reconstructing major defects of the lower eyelids.[4] The controversy as to the relative merits of these two procedures continues in the ophthalmic and plastic surgical literature and when the subject is discussed at scientific meetings. These two basic approaches will be discussed and illustrated. The relative merits of each procedure will be reviewed and following this, the author's philosophy on the use of these two methods will be presented.

Mustardé Technique for Reconstruction of Major Lower Eyelid Defects (Figure 55)

Mustardé's technique[3] consists of obtaining a composite nasal septal cartilage and mucosal graft through an intranasal operation, preserving the perichondrium and mucous membrane on the opposite side of the nasal septum to avoid a septal perforation. Once this graft has been obtained, it is necessary to trim the nasal cartilage down to a thickness of 2 mm or less. This must be done carefully and is necessary to prevent the reconstructed lower eyelid from being thick and unsightly. The mucous membrane is trimmed to fit the conjunctival defect. The cartilage is cut back from the edge of the mucous membrane so that there is a free edge of mucous membrane at the newly created lid margin. Once this composite graft has been properly trimmed to fit the defect, the septal cartilage is approximated to the remaining tarsus with long acting absorbable sutures burying the knots within the lid. The conjunctiva can be approximated to the mucous membrane of the nasal septum with knots buried within the substance of the lid. No suture material is allowed to touch the cornea. This graft provides an outstanding mucous secreting lining and replaces the missing tarsus. The graft can be made slightly less wide than the defect to give firm support to the reconstructed lower eyelid. Once this inner lining has been established, attention is turned to the outer lining, which is provided by a large rotation cheek flap. (This flap was previously described in Chapter 3.) The incision is carried backward and slightly upward from the lateral canthus and then horizontally back to the anterior temple hairline and tragus area and inferiorly just in front of the ear. The flap is elevated in the deep subcutaneous plane out onto the cheek and even into the neck, if necessary. To equalize the sides of the resulting donor site after the flap has been transferred, either a back cut on the flap itself or a Burow's triangle on the outer donor margin is required. (These techniques have previously been discussed and illustrated in Figures 18 and 19.)

After the flap has been rotated into place, it is vitally important to place one or two permanent sutures from the dermis of the flap to the periosteum above the lateral canthus at the orbital rim. This creates an upward pull on the flap to stabilize it and avoids the development of an ectropion. The flap is trimmed to fit the defect. A standing cone at the rotation point of the flap can be removed, if necessary. The flap is quite safe (if properly elevated) since it has a wide base. Dermal and skin closure are carried out on the donor site and on the medial edge of the flap. Fine sutures are used to approximate the mucous membrane of the inner lining to the skin of the outer lining. It is preferable to have the mucous membranes slightly higher than the skin layer to prevent skin from growing over the edge and possibly irritating the cornea. This technique is particularly useful for very large defects created by the excision of large cancers involving the entire lower lid and even a portion of the upper lid as illustrated in Figure 56. This defect was very nicely reconstructed with the technique of Mustardé. One of the objections that some ophthalmic plastic surgeons have to this technique is that even with extremely meticulous technique, a slight notch can develop at the margin of the lower eyelid (Figure 57).

Hughes Technique for Reconstruction of Major Lower Eyelid Defects (Figure 58)

The Hughes[2] technique utilizes a tarsoconjunctival flap from the undersurface of the upper eyelid, which is advanced to provide inner lining for the defect in the lower eyelid. At one time this technique fell into disrepute because the incision for the flap was made at the white line. This caused development of entropion and trichiasis in a great number of cases. The technique was modified, and it is now recommended that the inferior incision for the upper eyelid tarsoconjunctival flap always be made 4 to 5 mm above the lid margin to avoid these postoperative complications. The U-shaped incision based superiorly is carried through the conjunctival and tarsal layers. Careful dissection is carried out in the layer between the tarsus and the levator muscle back into the fornix of the superior eyelid conjunctiva. The flap is based on the conjunctiva and Muller's muscle. The flap is advanced into the lower eyelid and secured with sutures through the tarsus of the flap to the remaining tarsus of the lower eyelid. It is recommended that the flap be made approximately 25 percent less wide than the defect of the lower eyelid.

It is helpful to place a retention suture through the two lateral segments of the remaining lower eyelid to avoid having the lower eyelid defect appear larger than it actually is owing to retraction of the remaining segments. Once the flap is securely in place, outer lining is provided by a skin graft (Figure 58) or an inferiorly based advancement lower eyelid flap from the remaining eyelid tissues (Figure 59). The tarsoconjunctival flap is left in place for 4 to 8 weeks, and then a releasing procedure is carried out. In the releasing procedure the incision through the flap is made slightly beveled anteriorly so the mucous membrane side will be higher than the skin side of the remaining lower eyelid. This will prevent skin from growing over the edge of the newly created lower eyelid where it could come in contact with the cornea.

If the patient has an intrinsic disease of the eye, such as glaucoma, or a cornea that requires frequent drops or medications, this flap may be contraindicated. It may also be contraindicated in the patient in whom the involved lid is in an only seeing eye. The patient must be willing to have the involved eyelid shut for a period of 4 to 6 weeks before the releasing procedure is carried out.

Discussion

When there is a moderate to large full thickness defect of the lower eyelid involving the margin of the lid and up to 8 to 10 mm in vertical height, the Hughes technique is probably the preferred method of reconstruction if the patient has a normal upper eyelid and no intrinsic eye disease on that side. The Mustardé technique is indicated in patients in whom tissue of the opposing lid is unavailable and in those with advanced cancers, which require more tissue for satisfactory reconstruction than can be obtained from the opposite lid (Figure 55). This technique is also indicated if the tumor and resulting defect extends down below the eyelid and is large in the vertical direction.

The objectional complications of entropion and trichiasis found with the earlier Hughes technique procedures have been obviated by the modification of leaving 4 to 5 mm of normal tarsus of the lower margin of the upper eyelid. Notching of the lower eyelids has been a problem with the Mustardé technique. Experience in ophthalmic plastic surgery and a thorough knowledge of eyelid anatomy are required to obtain good results using the tarsoconjunctival flap (Hughes) technique. For this reason, the Mustardé technique has appealed to plastic surgeons with little experience in ophthalmic plastic surgery. A facial plastic surgeon embarking upon the reconstruction of major full thickness defects of the lower eyelid should have a thorough understanding of both of these techniques, and knowledge and judgment as to their relative merits.

Reconstruction of Medial Canthal Defects

Flap reconstructions in the medial canthal area have previously been dealt with by the author.[5] On the nasal side of the medial canthal region, glabellar flaps (Chapter 4) for smaller defects and forehead flaps (Chapter 9) for larger defects are usually utilized. The reader is referred to this previous work[5] and Chapters 4 and 5 of this book for more information on this subject.

REFERENCES

1. Anderson RL, Hatt MN, Dixon R: Medial ectropion—a new technique. Arch Ophthalmol 97:521–524, 1978
2. Hughes WL: New method for rebuilding lower lid. Arch Ophthalmol 17:1008, 1937
3. Mustardé JC: Repair and Reconstruction in the Orbital Region. A Practical Guide. Baltimore: The Williams & Wilkins Co., 1966
4. Converse JA (ed): Reconstructive Plastic Surgery, 2nd ed. Philadelphia London Toronto: WB Saunders, 1977, pp. 882–902
5. Becker FF: Reconstructive surgery of the medial canthal region. Ann Plast Surg 7:259–268, 1981

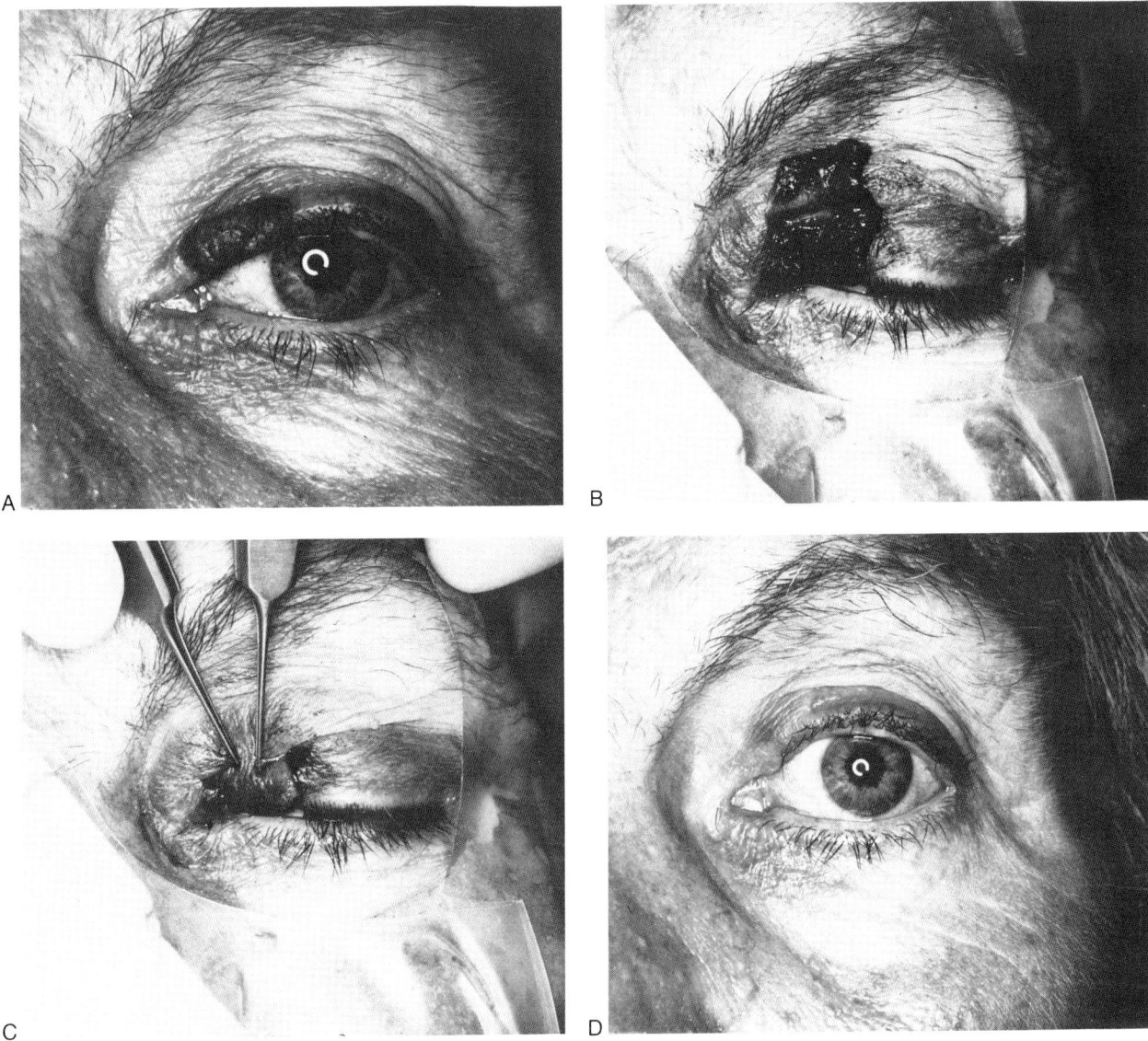

Figure 49. A, Large seborrheic keratosis of left upper eyelid involving the lid margin. B, Tumor excised, advancement flap elevated. C, Flap advanced to cover skin defect of lid. D, Final result, four months postoperative.

84 Facial Reconstruction with Local and Regional Flaps

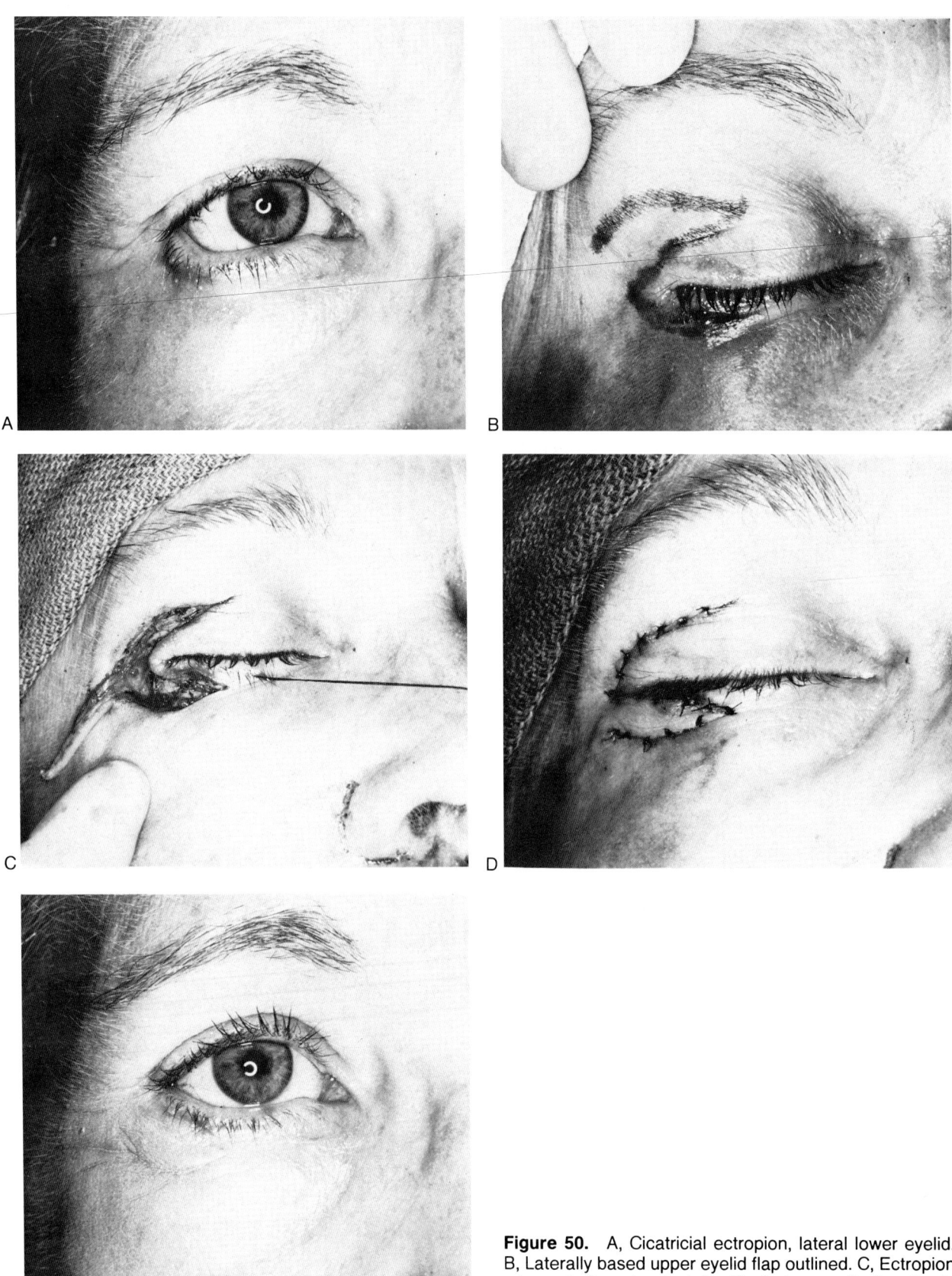

Figure 50. A, Cicatricial ectropion, lateral lower eyelid. B, Laterally based upper eyelid flap outlined. C, Ectropion released, flap elevated. D, Final closure. E, Result, six months postoperative.

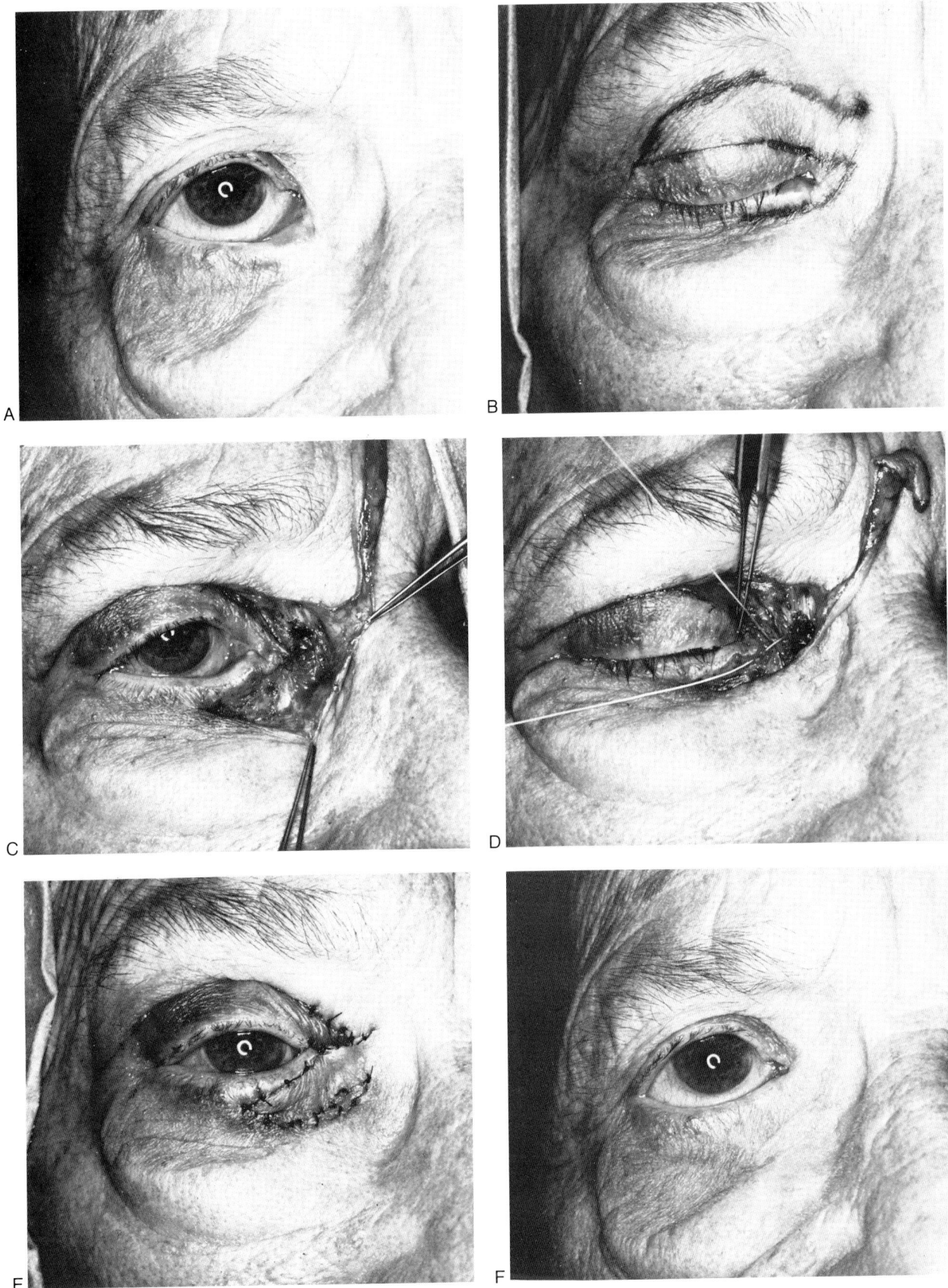

Figure 51. A, Cicatricial ectropion, medial aspect of lower eyelid; previous attempt at correction by another surgeon failed. B, Medially based upper eyelid flap outlined. C, Ectropion released, flap elevated. D, Lower crus of medial canthal tendon plicated. E, Final closure. F, Result, nine months postoperative.

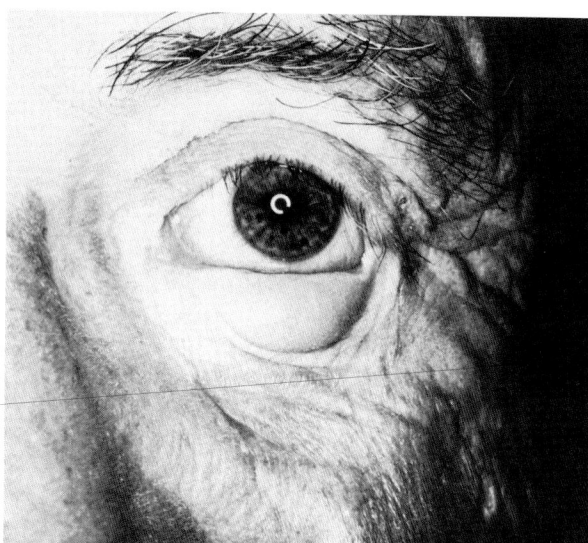

Figure 52. Lower eyelid previously reconstructed with a midline forehead flap by another surgeon. Note marked thickening of lower eyelid.

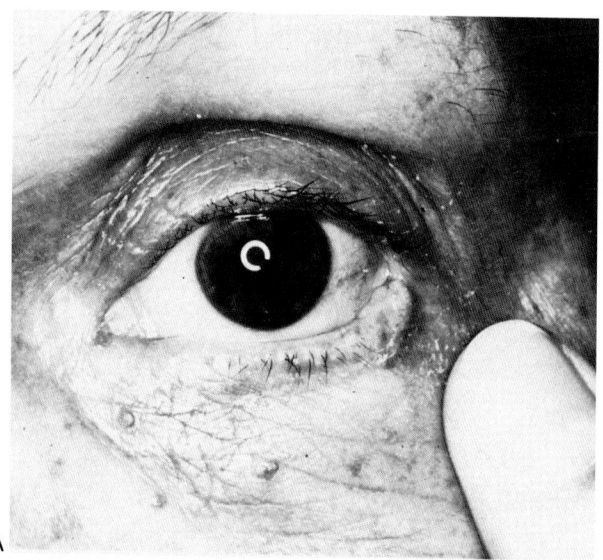
A

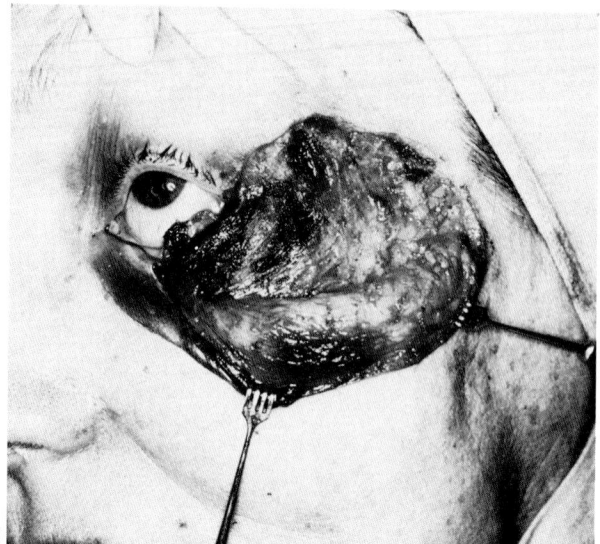
B

Figure 53. A, Basal cell carcinoma of lateral lower eyelid margin involving all layers. B, Tumor excised, cheek flap elevated.

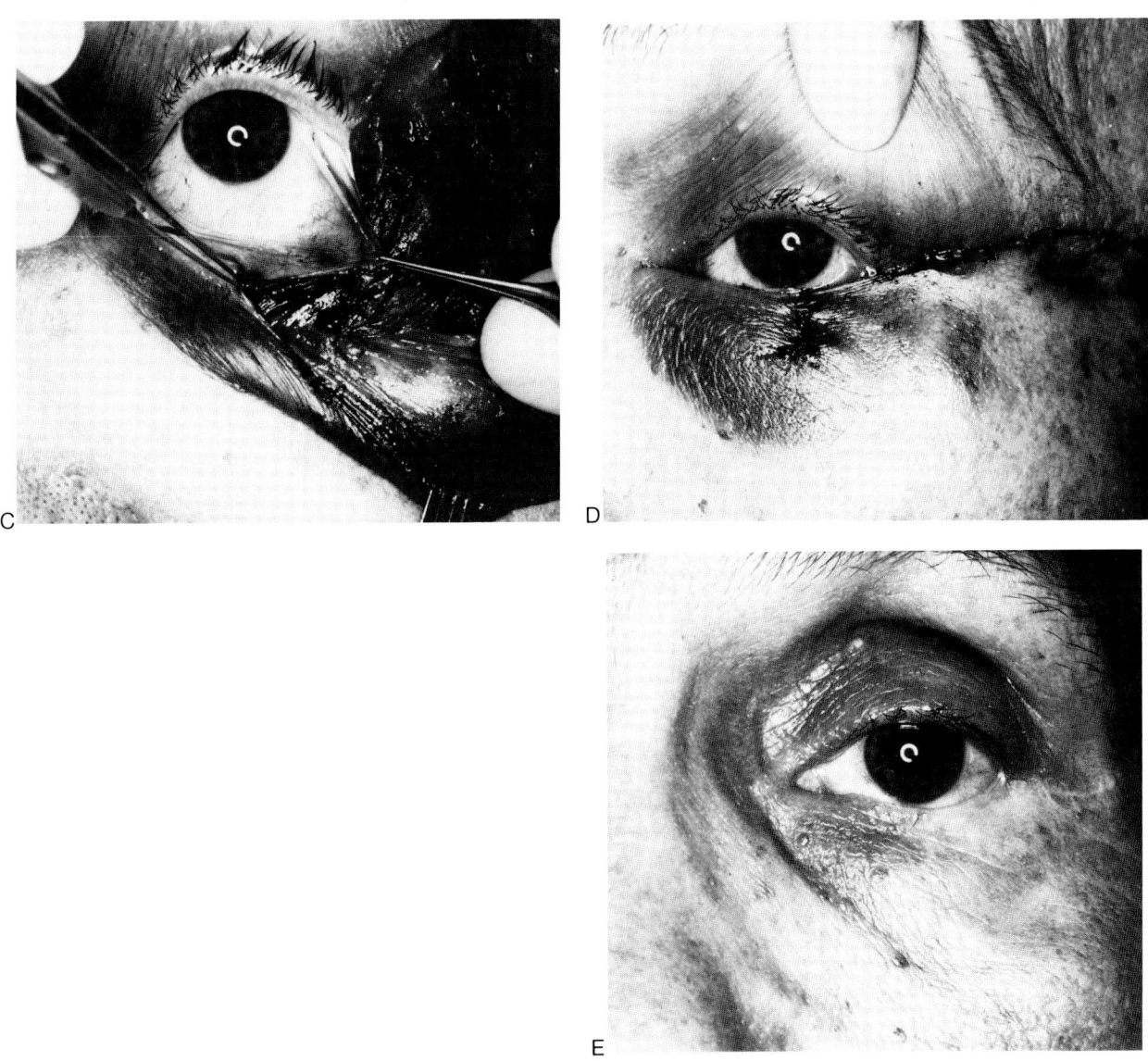

Figure 53. (cont.) C, Conjunctival flap from lower fornix elevated and advanced for closure of inner lining. D, Final closure. E, Result, six months postoperative.

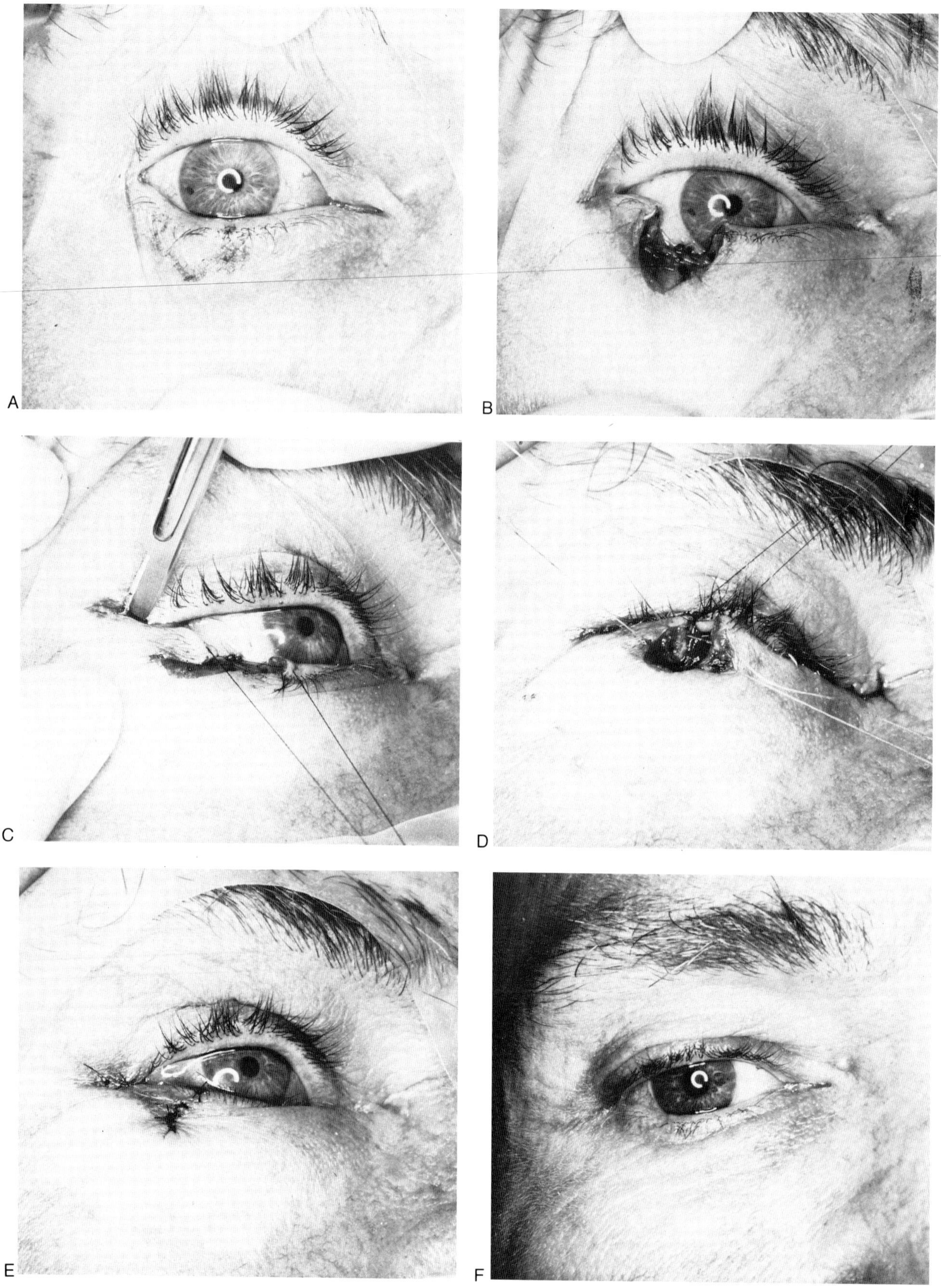

Figure 54. A, Basal cell carcinoma of lower eyelid margin, pentagonal excision outlined. B, Tumor excised. C, Lateral cantholysis with division of lower crus of lateral canthal tendon. D, Tarsal layer closure. E, Final closure. F, Result, six months postoperative.

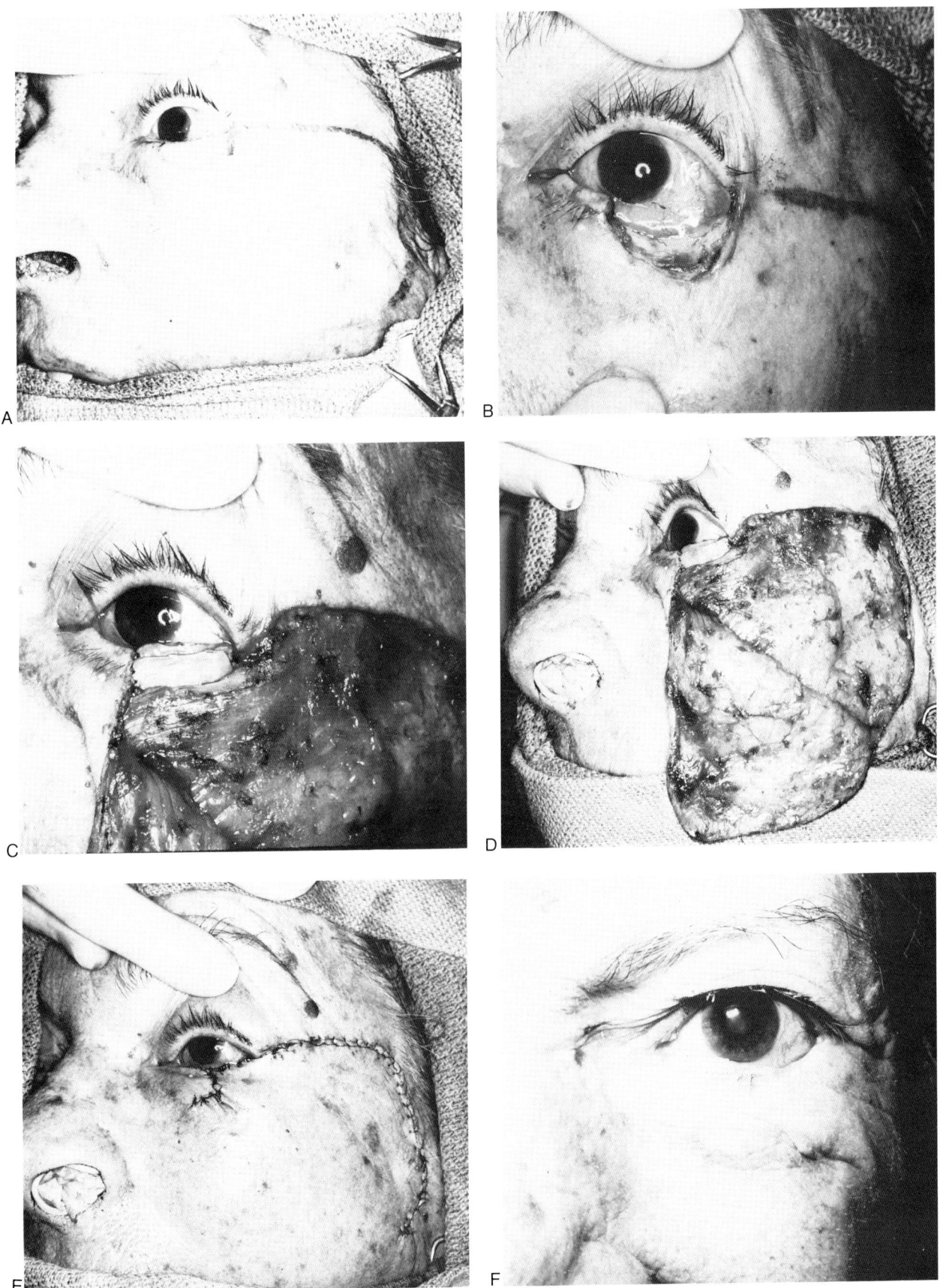

Figure 55. A, Large basal cell carcinoma involving margin of lower eyelid; Mustardé flap outlined. B, Tumor excised. C, Cartilage-mucosal composite graft from nasal septum sutured into place for inner lining. D, Flap elevated. E, Final closure. F, Result, four months postoperative.

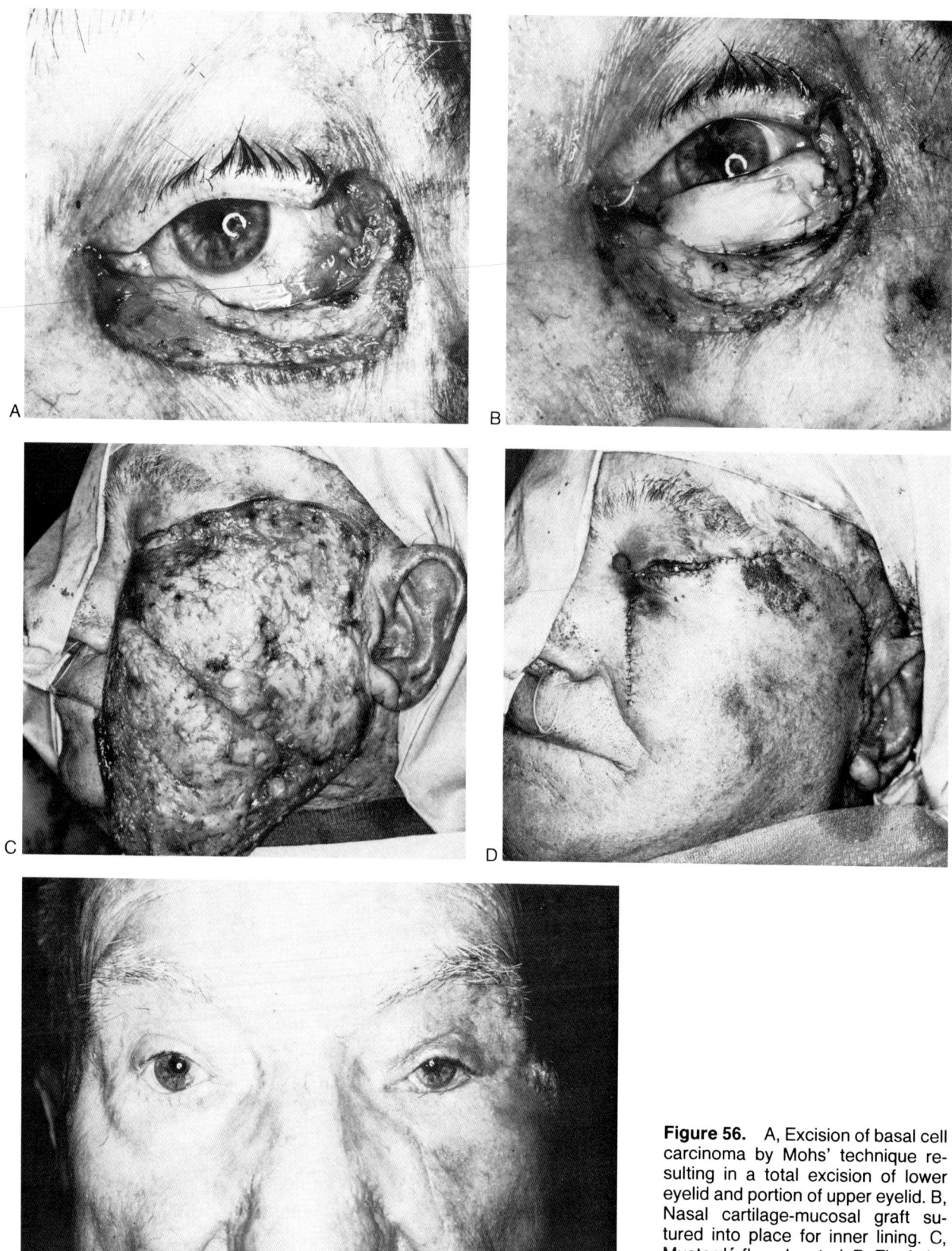

Figure 56. A, Excision of basal cell carcinoma by Mohs' technique resulting in a total excision of lower eyelid and portion of upper eyelid. B, Nasal cartilage-mucosal graft sutured into place for inner lining. C, Mustardé flap elevated. D, Final closure. E, Final result, three months postoperative.

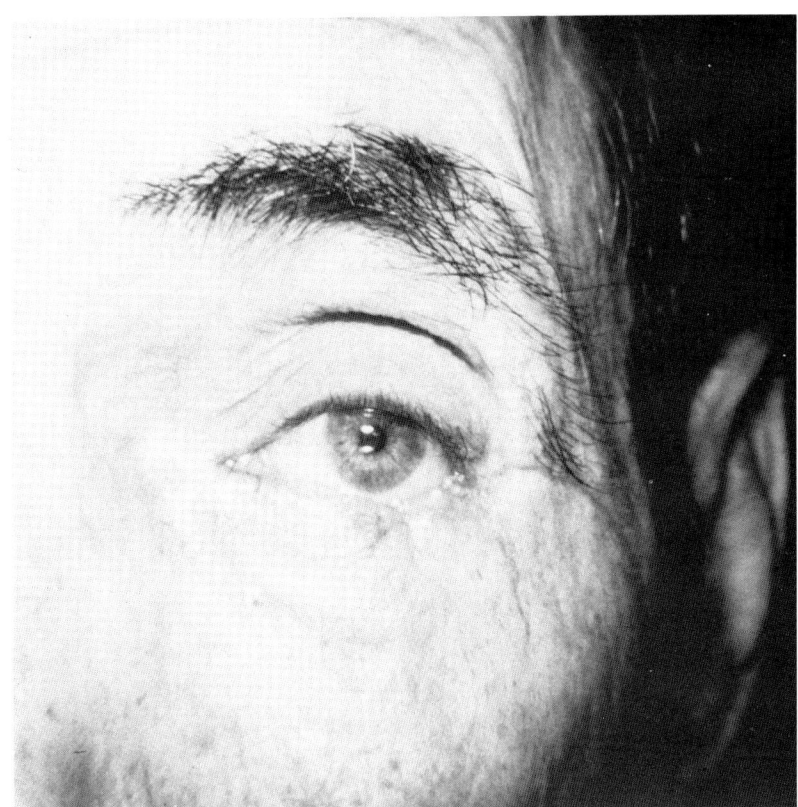

Figure 57. Postoperative Mustardé flap reconstruction of full thickness lower eyelid defect with small notch of lower eyelid.

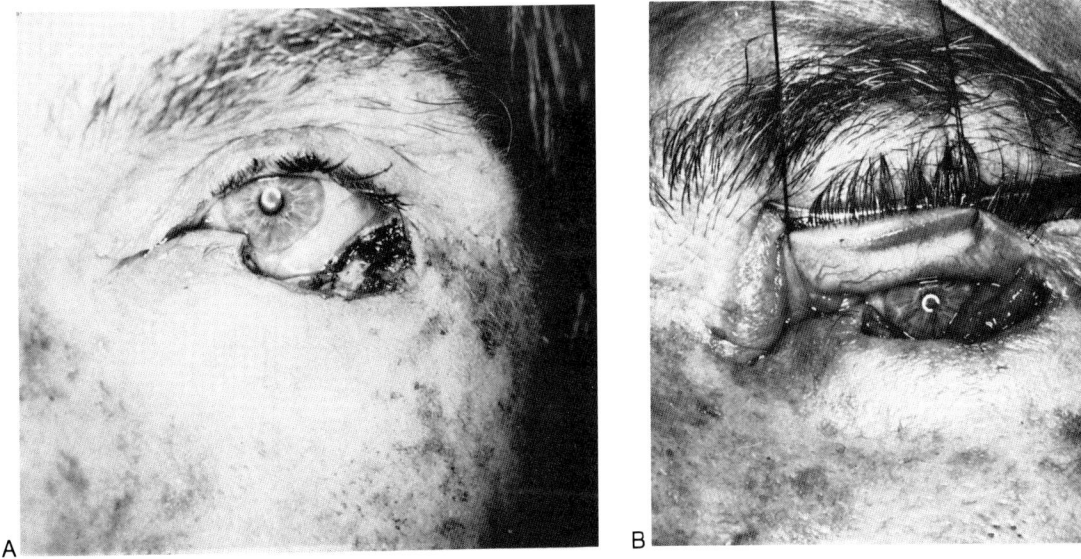

Figure 58. A, Full thickness defect of lower eyelid involving three-quarters of lower eyelid secondary to excision of marginal basal cell carcinoma by Mohs' technique. B, Upper eyelid everted; note tarsus.

92 Facial Reconstruction with Local and Regional Flaps

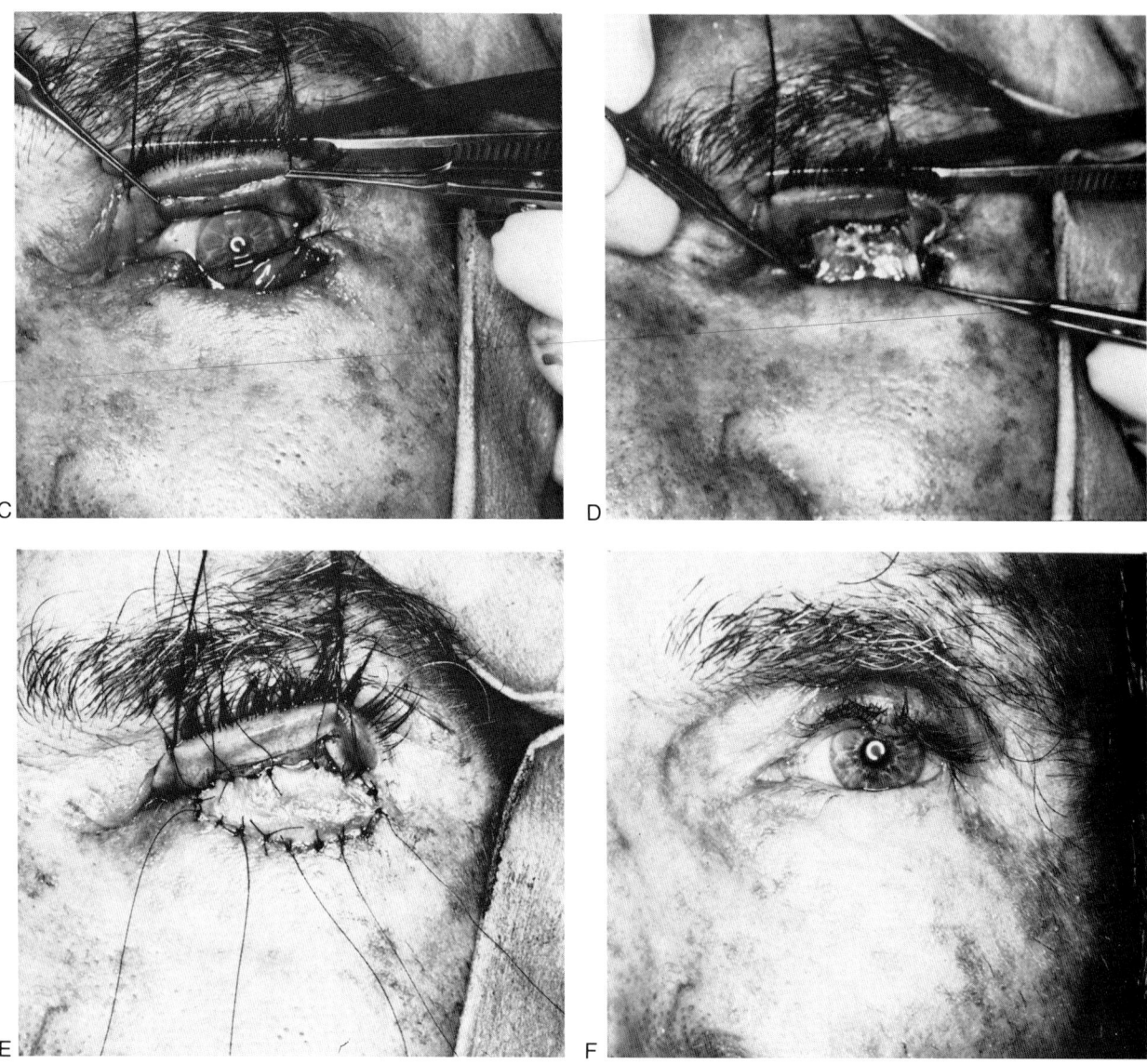

Figure 58. (cont.) C, Incision for tarsoconjunctival flap carried out 4 mm above lower tarsal border. Note retention suture in lower eyelid. D, Flap advanced into lower eyelid defect for inner lining. E, Full thickness skin graft applied to flap for outer lining. F, Final result, one year following releasing procedure.

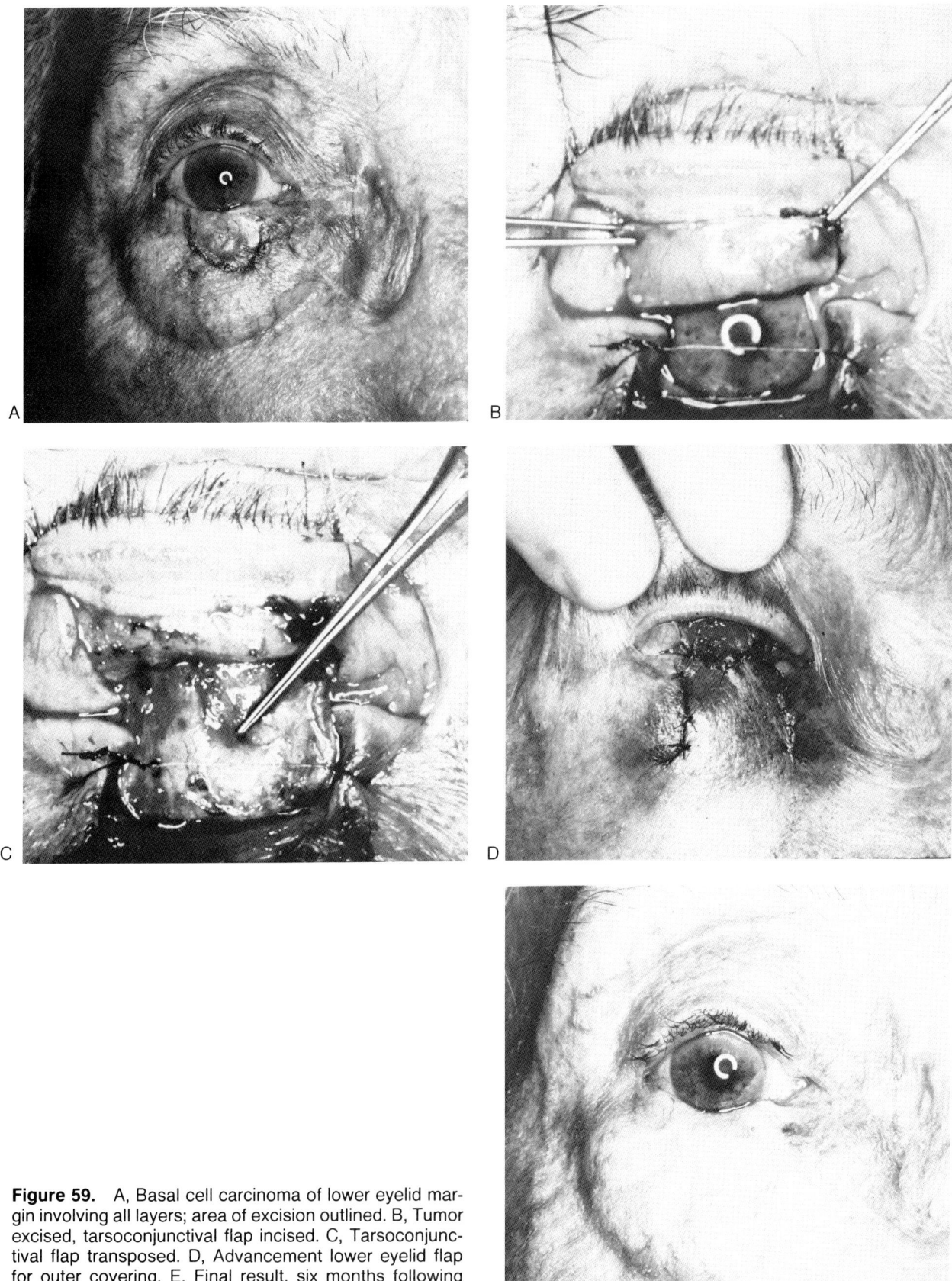

Figure 59. A, Basal cell carcinoma of lower eyelid margin involving all layers; area of excision outlined. B, Tumor excised, tarsoconjunctival flap incised. C, Tarsoconjunctival flap transposed. D, Advancement lower eyelid flap for outer covering. E, Final result, six months following releasing procedure.

9 Forehead Flaps

The earliest descriptions of facial reconstruction with flaps were from ancient India during the Vedic times (2000 B.C.–500 B.C.).[1] These reconstructions involved the use of the vertical midline forehead flap for nasal reconstruction. The punishment for the crime of adultery in ancient India was amputation of the nose. During those times, the Koomas, who were members of a cast of tile makers or potters, developed the art of reconstructing these destroyed noses. This procedure is often referred to even now as the Indian method of reconstructive rhinoplasty. Musculocutaneous (myocutaneous) flaps have been popularized within the last several years and often are referred to as new techniques. The midline forehead flap is a musculocutaneous flap that has been used since many centuries before Christ. This technique had a resurgence of interest in Italy in the 15th century and then fell into disrepute for another two centuries. Interest in subtotal nasal reconstruction with forehead flaps was revitalized in 19th century Europe and was used in various forms by French and particularly German surgeons during the mid-19th and early 20th centuries. Many variations of the midline forehead flap have been described, such as the oblique, up and down, sickle, sea gull; however, the vertical midline forehead flap with its variations is still the workhorse flap for subtotal nasal reconstruction.

In the early 1960's, McGregor[2] popularized the use of the horizontal forehead flap for intraoral and facial reconstruction. This flap enjoyed great popularity in major head and neck reconstructive efforts during the 1960's and into the late 1970's. Although the technique was well worked out and the success rate was excellent, the resulting grafted forehead deformity was often unsightly (Figure 60). The use of musculocutaneous flaps from distant sites in the reconstruction of major head and neck deformities has made the horizontal forehead flap relatively obsolete.

The major emphasis in this chapter will be on describing the midline forehead flap and the technical details in its execution. A brief discussion at the end of this chapter will concern the island forehead flap, which is a less reliable variant. Chapter 10 will deal with major facial reconstructions with multiple flaps. It will be necessary for the reader to assimilate the material contained in both these chapters to get the maximum information on the uses of the midline forehead flap.

MIDLINE FOREHEAD FLAP

The midline forehead flap is probably the only facial flap that derives its blood supply from both the internal and external carotid artery systems. The major blood supply for this flap is from the paired supratrochlear arteries, which anastamose with their ipsilateral supraorbital arteries. Collateral circulation connects the supratrochlear artery systems. These arterial supplies are terminal branches of the ophthalmic artery in the internal carotid artery system. The branches of these arteries richly anastamose with the terminal branches of the angular artery, which is a terminal artery of the facial artery, a branch of the external carotid artery system. Therefore, this flap has two blood supplies: an axial pattern supply from the supratrochlear arteries (internal carotid system) and a random pattern supply from branches of the facial artery (external carotid system). The richness of the vascular supply in this area is probably the reason that this is one of the most reliable facial flaps that has ever been devised. This flap has stood the test of time of many centuries of ancient and modern history. Loss of any skin of a midline forehead flap has never been seen by the author.

The flap is primarily used in subtotal nasal reconstruction and partial cheek reconstruction. The flap can even be harvested from the forehead on more than one occasion, and four patients who had reharvesting of vertical midline forehead flaps for additional reconstruction procedures of the nose were reported by Conley and Price in 1981.[3]

Technique (Figure 61)

A vertical flap is outlined using two parallel lines from the root of the nose to the hairline and connected by a horizontal limb at the hairline. A width of 2.5 cm is recommended at the root of the nose, and this may be widened to 3.5 cm near the hairline. Various oblique or horizontal extensions can be made at the superior aspect of the forehead depending on the nature of the nasal or facial deformity to be reconstructed.

A piece of gauze is stretched between the base of the flap at its rotation point and out to the end of the flap. The distal end of this gauze is brought inferiorly to be sure the flap will reach the proposed defect. Local anesthetic containing a vasoconstrictor is injected surrounding the previously marked areas and out into the lateral forehead in the subgaleal plane as well as into the donor site. This local anesthetic is employed even if general anesthesia is being used on the patient. The donor area is prepared or cleared of tumor as is indicated by the nature of the disease. Incisions are made in the superior aspect of the flap through skin and soft tissues including the galea down to the periosteum. The incisions are made through these layers down to near the root of the nose, where the incisions are made more superficially to avoid damage to the supratrochlear vessels. Dissection is carried out in the subgaleal plane superficial to the periosteum down to the root of the nose. Careful scissor and blunt dissection is used in the lateral area of the flap at the root of the nose to avoid interruption of the vascular pedicles. To rotate the flap, it may be necessary to cut through this pedicle on one side of the flap, although this is not always the case. Dissection is then carried out laterally in the forehead defect in the subgaleal plane as far as is necessary to allow the forehead to close in the midline. Often vertical relaxing incisions are made very superficially through the galea with a light cutting cautery to aid this closure. The forehead incision is closed with heavy sutures on the galeal layer, absorbable sutures on the dermal layer, and fine sutures on the skin layer. The flap is transposed into the defect, trimmed to fit the defect, and sutured into place appropriately.

Since the neural innervation of the frontalis muscle approaches laterally, there is no significant interference with frontalis function from this procedure. The dissection of the forehead is carried out in the deep plane below the level of the supraorbital neurovascular bundles, and therefore sensory innervation of the forehead is undisturbed. Although the vertical forehead closure crosses the lines of relaxed skin tension, this incision heals remarkably well with an excellent aesthetic result in most cases.

The pedicle of the flap is divided about three weeks after the primary procedure (Figure 62E, F). The unused portion of the forehead flap is amputated and not replaced on the forehead. This gives a more favorable cosmetic result than replacing the unused portion of the forehead flap back on the forehead (Figure 76). If the medial ends of the eyebrows were brought close together during the initial procedure, this can be corrected with a portion of the base of the unused flap during the secondary releasing procedure. A wide defect of the forehead that cannot be closed primarily can be closed by extending horizontal incisions at the superior aspect of the forehead defect laterally into the scalp and rotating the flaps in to close the defect. This flap is an excellent method to close large, deep medial canthal defects (Figure 61), defects involving the skin of the entire nasal dorsum (Figure 62), and nasal ala defects (Figure 63). These flaps tend to remain thick for several months following surgery owing to lymphedema. If this problem does not correct itself with time, debulking procedures and scar revisions are usually quite helpful in improving the aesthetic appearance.

ISLAND FOREHEAD FLAP

In 1963, Converse and Wood-Smith[4] reported their experience with the midline island forehead flap based on a subcutaneous pedicle containing the supratrochlear artery and vein. This procedure has the distinct advantage of being a one stage operation that avoids the unsightly skin pedicle which is necessary temporarily with the previous procedure.

The flap can be rotated into position either through a tunnel or directly through a vertical incision between the island and the recipient area on the nose with elevation of the skin off the pedicle. This flap has greater mobility than the usual vertical midline forehead flap because the subcutaneous pedicle is more mobile. The principle disadvantage of the island forehead flap is that it has one source of blood supply from the supratrochlear artery of the internal carotid artery system, and thus lacks the additional random pattern blood supply from the external carotid artery system that the midline verticle forehead flap enjoys. An additional disadvantage is the protrusion that may remain at the root of the nose as a result of the presence of the subcutaneous pedicle. This protrusion tends to regress with time. Because of vascular problems encountered with this flap (Figure 87), it is not recommended for routine use and it should only be employed by an experienced facial surgeon.

Technique (Figure 64)

A flap of appropriate size to reconstruct the defect is marked over the forehead in an inverted pattern. It is marked with a pedicle long enough to allow it to extend to the defect when elevated. A V-shaped portion of skin just above and below the flap can be excised to assist in the closure of the forehead defect. Local anesthetic is used in the forehead and the donor site as previously described. The defect is prepared or created. An incision is made at the superior aspect of the flap to the periosteal layer and it is dissected in the subgaleal plane as previously described. In the lower portion of the incision for the flap, the incision is made just through the skin. Either a tunnel is created in the subcutaneous plane from this point down into the defect, or an incision is made from the inferior aspect of the donor site to the defect to be reconstructed, and the skin is elevated laterally in the subcutaneous plane. A subcutaneous and muscular pedicle containing the supratrochlear artery and vein is then developed on one side. It is wise to keep this pedicle as wide as is feasible. The flap is rotated 180° into the defect. Great care is taken to avoid twisting or the pedicle. The forehead is closed in a manner similar to that for the midline forehead flap and the island skin paddle is sutured into the defect appropriately.

DISCUSSION

This chapter has dealt primarily with the technique and several of the applications of the midline forehead flap procedure. The next chapter will demonstrate how this very useful, versatile, and proven flap can be combined with other flaps in major nasal and facial reconstructions.

REFERENCES

1. Converse JA (ed): Reconstructive Plastic Surgery, 2nd ed. Philadelphia London Toronto: WB Saunders, 1977
2. McGregor IA: The temporal flap in intra-oral cancer—Its use in repairing the post-excisional defect. Br J Plast Surg 16:318, 1963
3. Conley JJ, Price JC: The midline vertical forehead flap. Otolaryngol Head Neck Surg 89:38–44, 1981
4. Converse JM, Wood-Smith D: Experiences with the forehead island flap with a subcutaneous pedicle. Plast Reconstr Surg 31:521–525, 1963

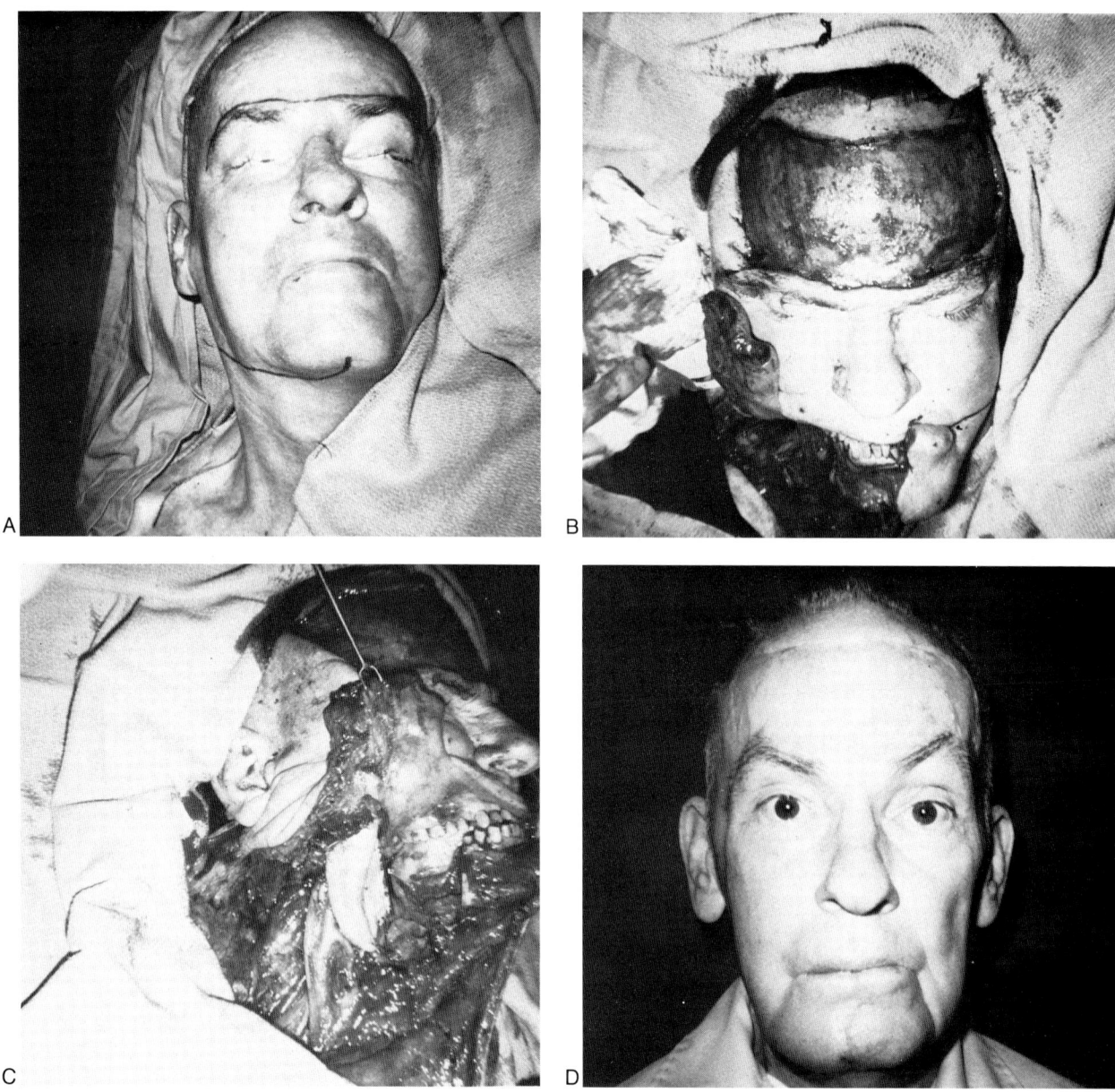

Figure 60. A, Horizontal forehead flap marked for major head and neck reconstruction. B, Forehead flap tunneled under zygoma into mouth. C, Flap in place for intraoral reconstruction following composite resection. D, Final result, note significant forehead deformity.

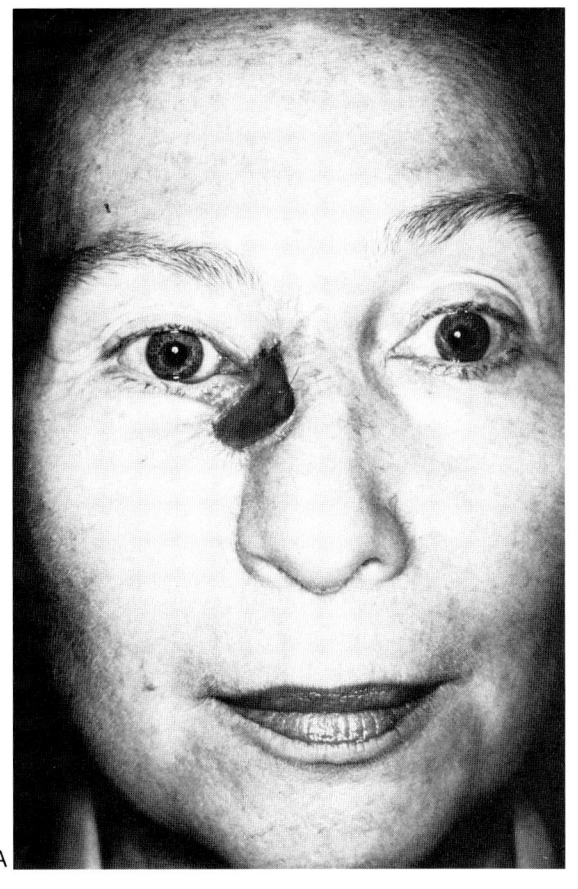
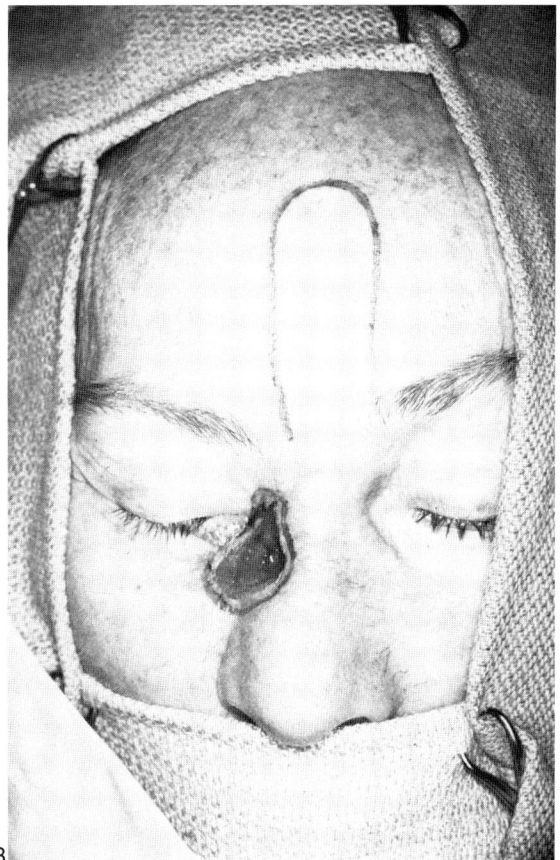
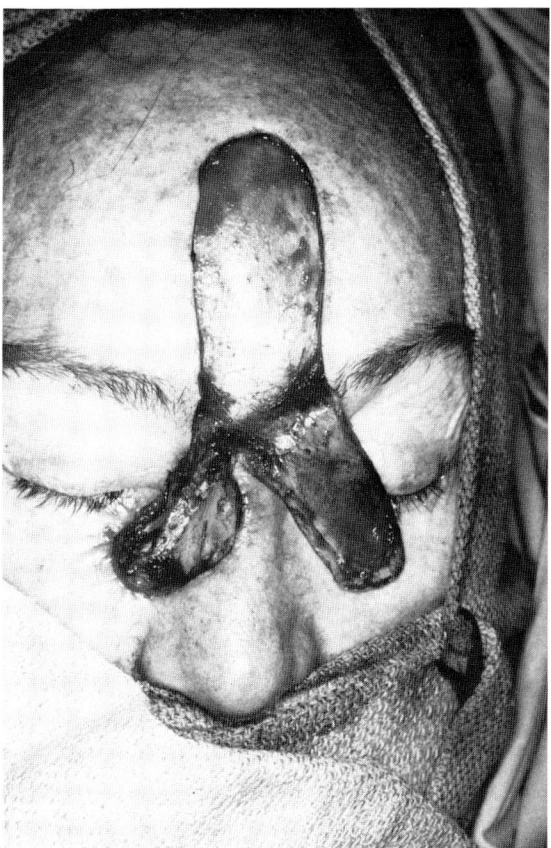

Figure 61. A, Large defect of right medial canthus one month following microscopically controlled excision of recurrent basal cell carcinoma by Dr. Fredric Mohs. Note early ectropion and downward displacement of medial aspect of right brow. B, Midline forehead flap outlined. C, Granulation and scar tissue removed, forehead flap elevated.

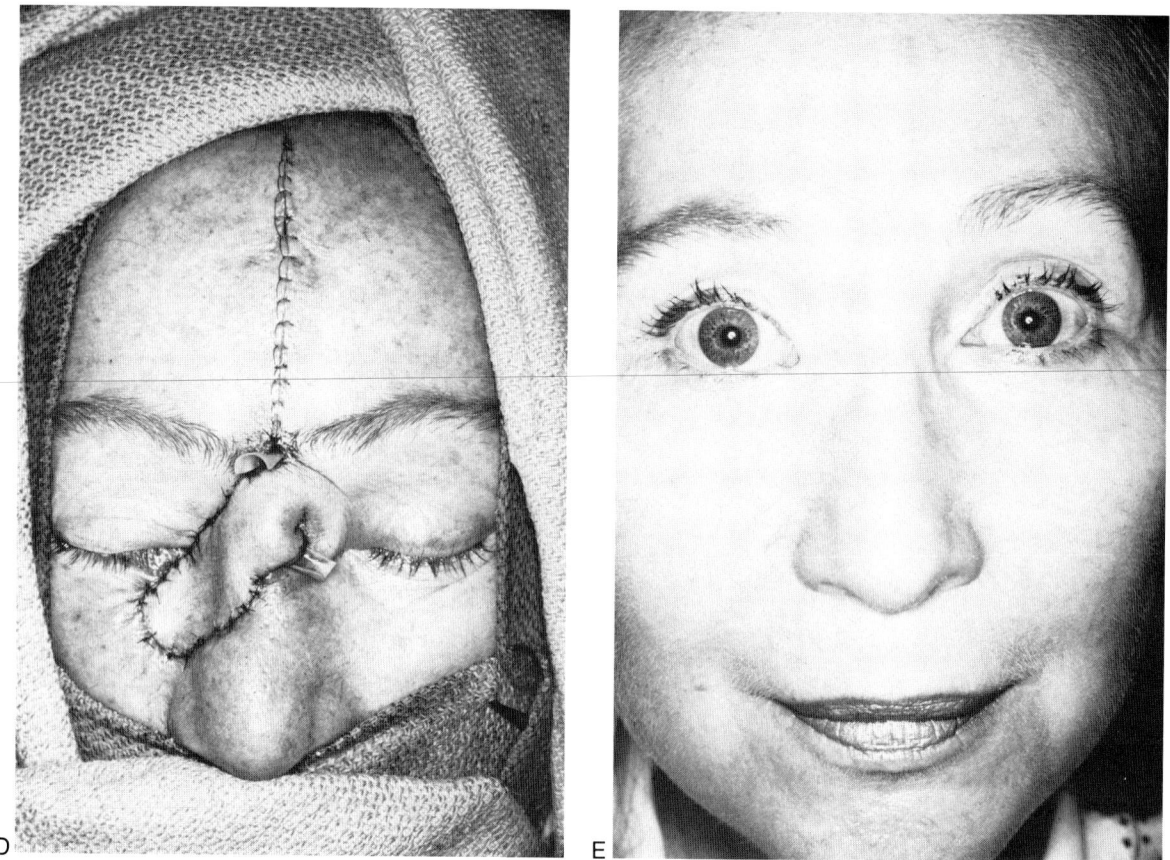

Figure 61 (cont.) D, Flap rotated into place, donor site closed in midline. E, Final result, one year postoperative. (Reprinted with permission from: Becker FF: Reconstructive surgery of medial canthal region. Ann Plast Surg 7:264–265, 1981)

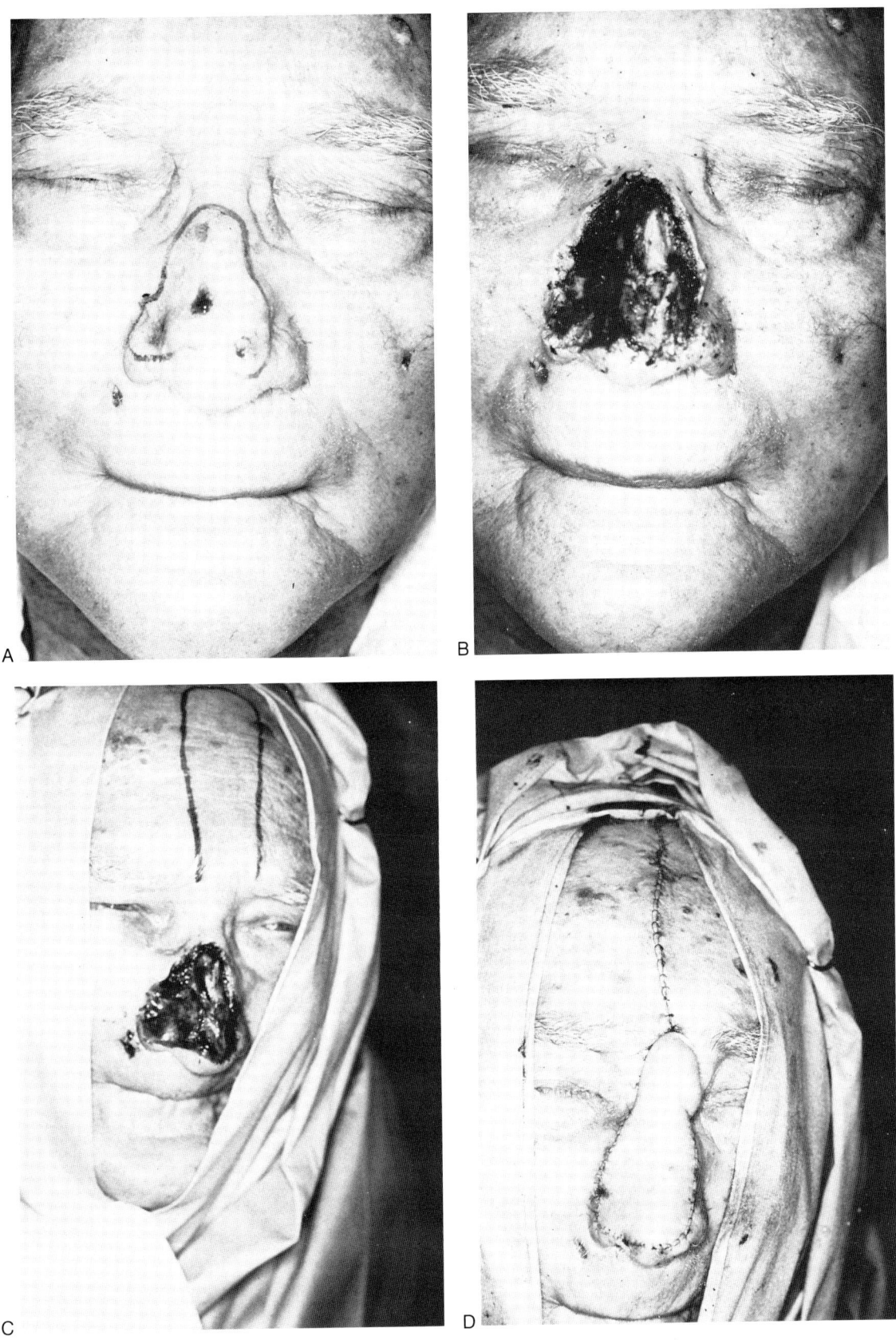

Figure 62. A, Multifocal recurrent basal cell carcinoma of entire dorsum of nose. B, Defect of skin of entire dorsum of nose including some cartilage and bone following Mohs' surgery. C, Midline forehead flap outlined. D, Flap rotated into place, donor site closed in midline.

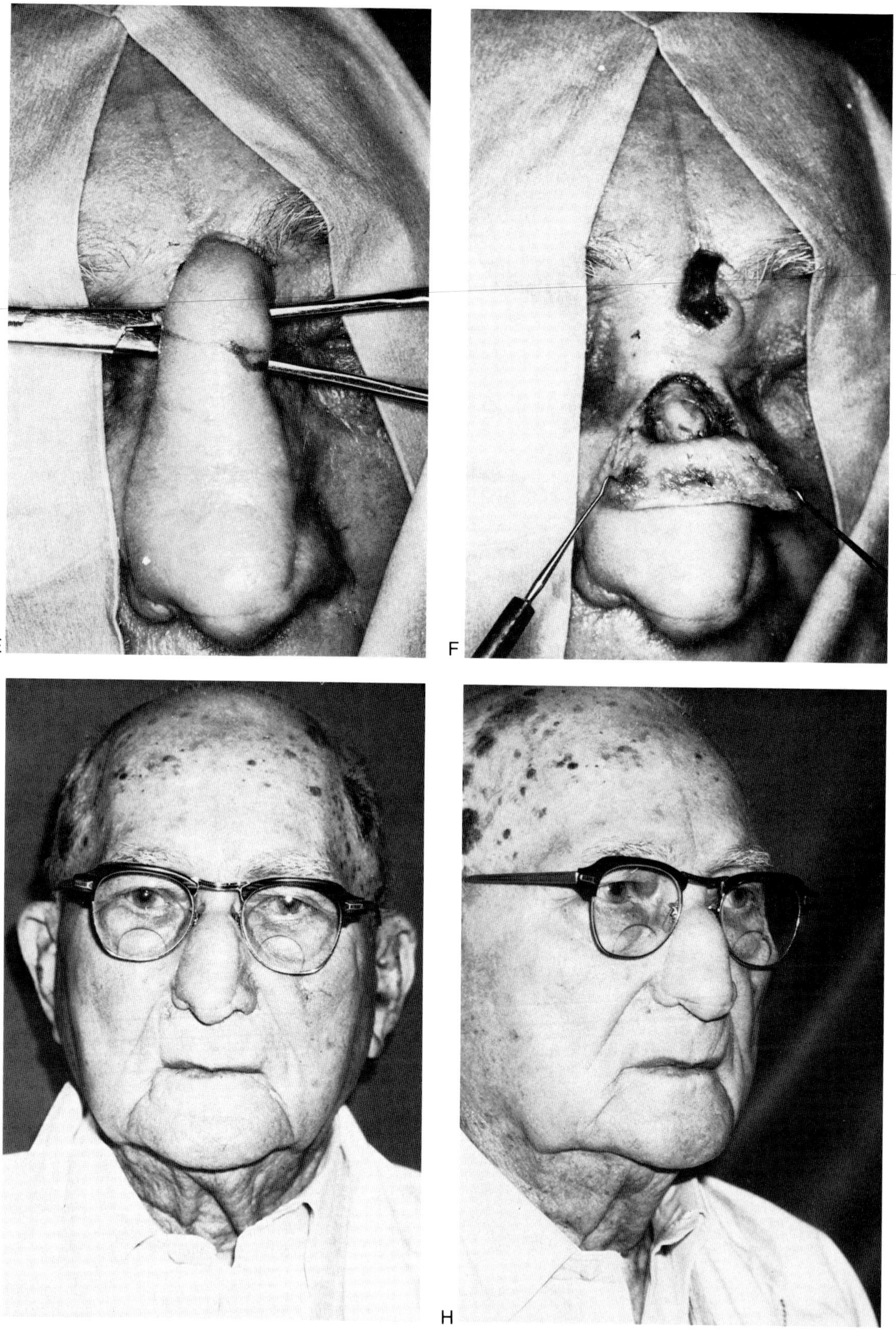

Figure 62. (cont.) E, Hemostat under pedicle of flap in preparation for division three weeks following primary procedure. F, Superior aspect of flap debulked, excess skin trimmed. G, Final result, three months postoperative, frontal view. H, Final result, three months postoperative, lateral view.

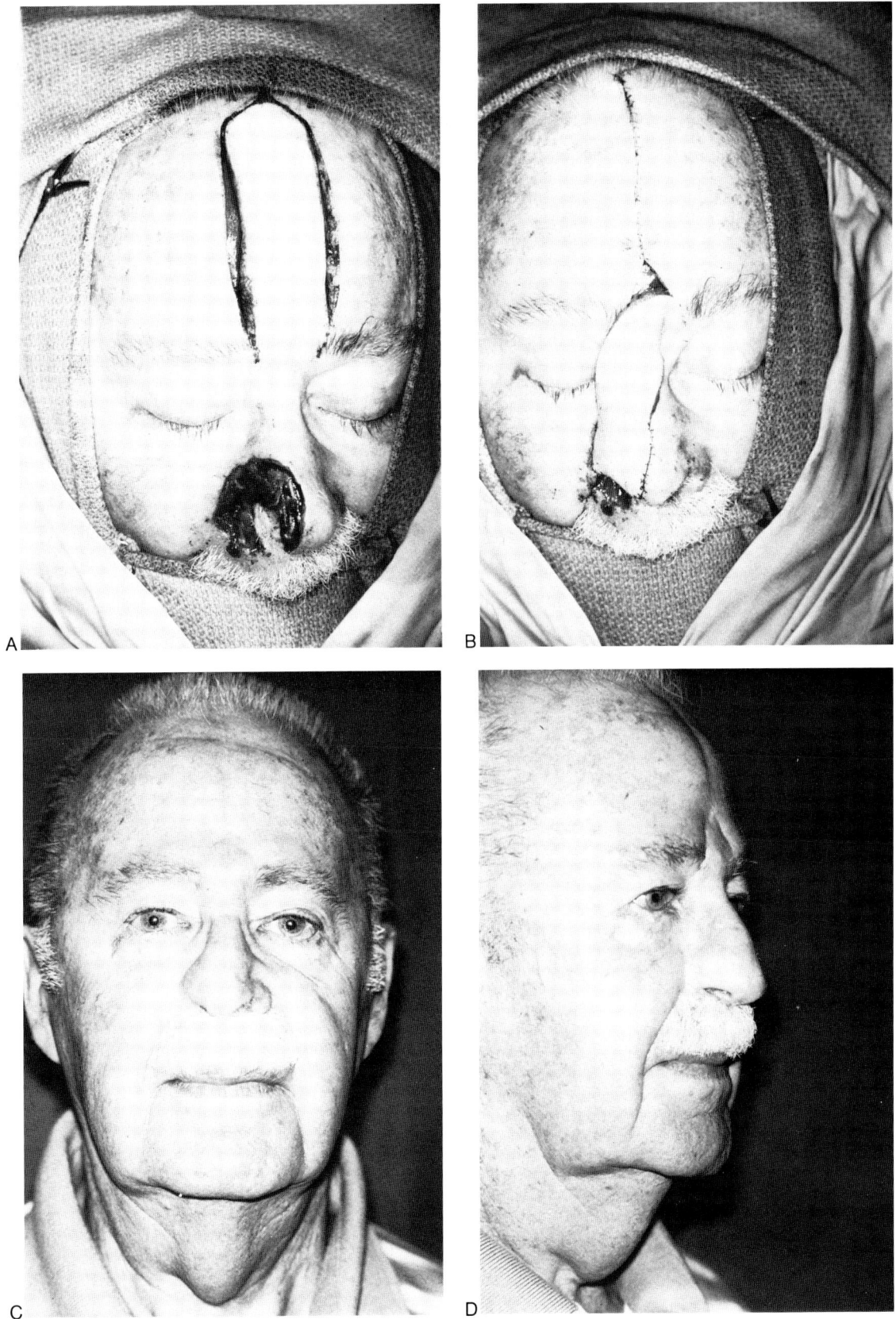

Figure 63. A, Large full thickness right nasal ala defect secondary to excision of sclerosing basal cell carcinoma by Mohs' technique, midline forehead flap elevated. B, Flap rotated into place, donor site closed primarily. C, Result, six months postoperative, frontal view. D, Result, six months postoperative, lateral view.

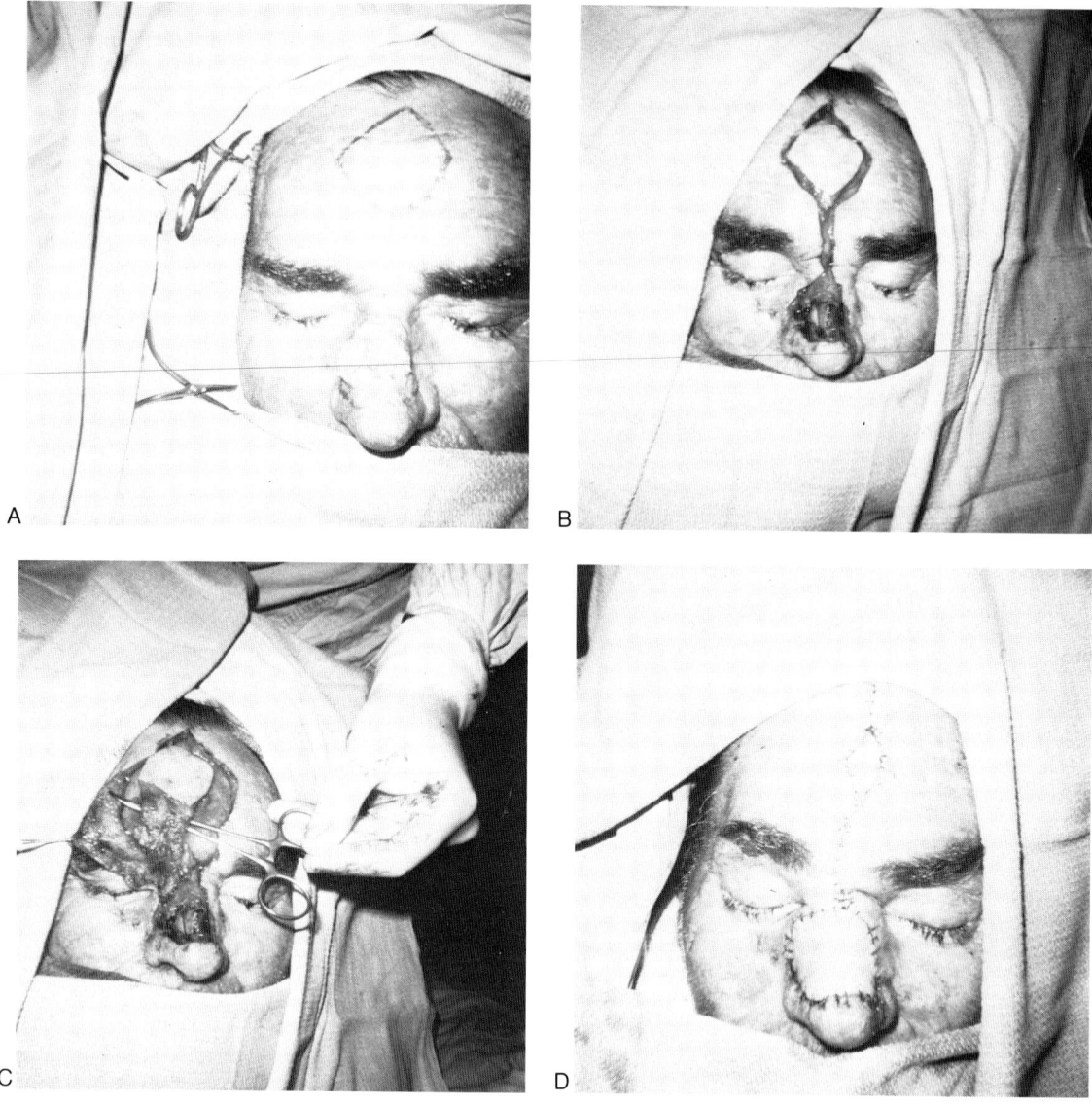

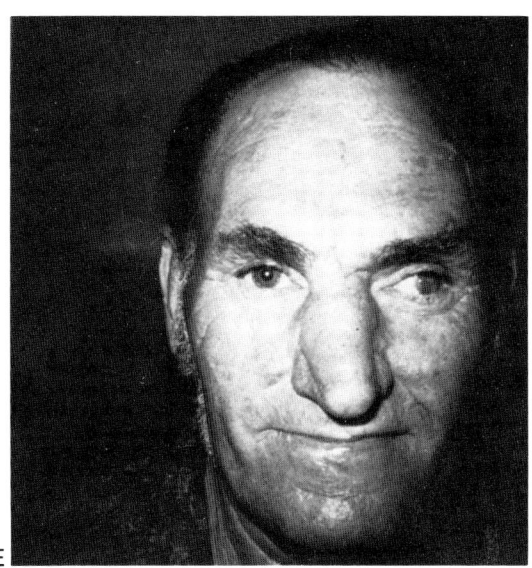

Figure 64. A, Excision of large squamous cell carcinoma of nasal dorsum outlined, island forehead flap designed. B, Tumor excised including cartilage and bone, flap elevated. C, Flap pedicled on supratrochlear artery and vein demonstrated. D, Final closure. E, Final result, nine months postoperative following dermabrasion of edges of flap. (Reprinted with permission from: Becker FF: Local tissue flaps in reconstructive facial plastic surgery. South Med J 70:677–680, 1977)

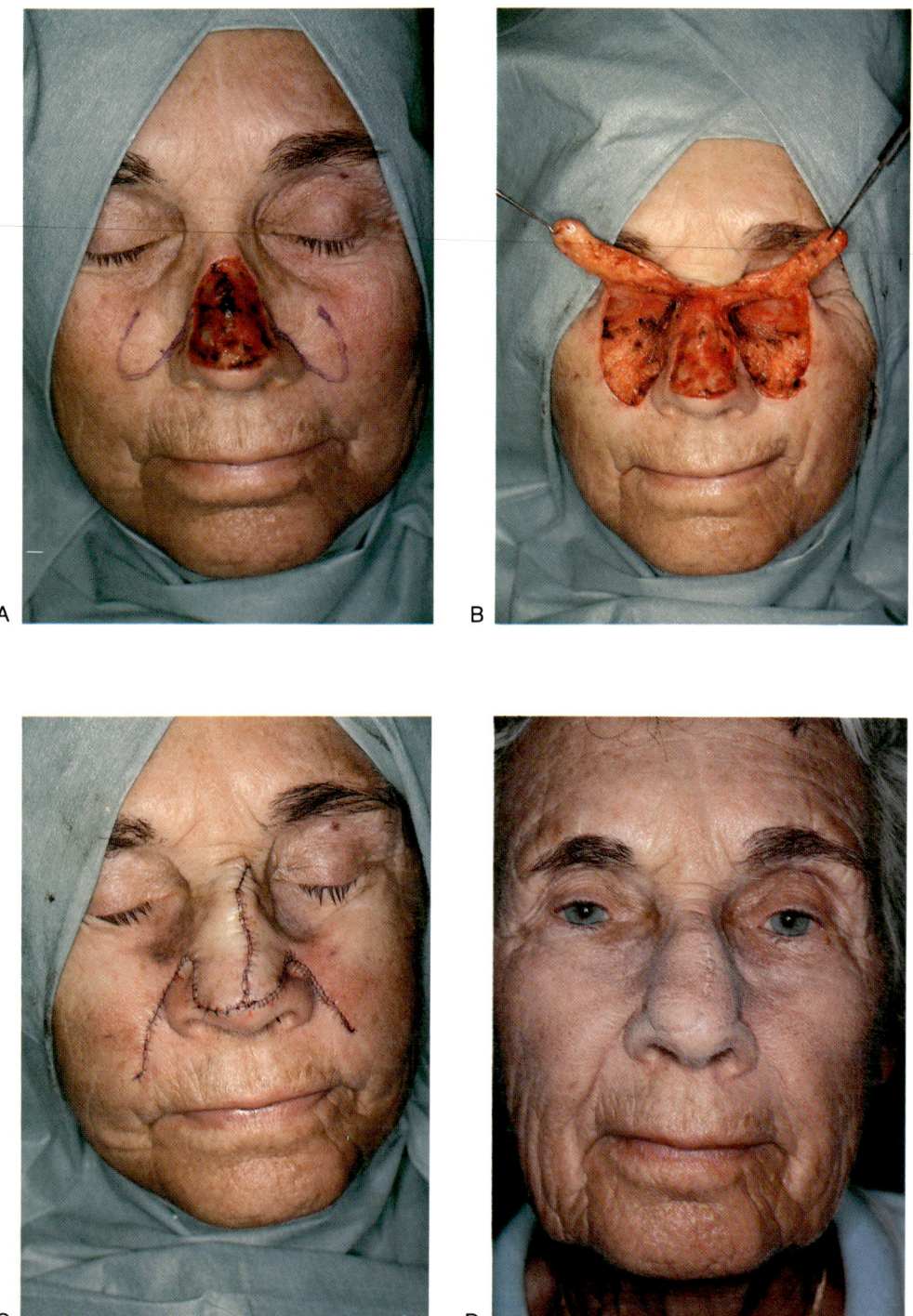

Color Plate I. Nasal defect created by microscopically controlled excision by the Mohs' technique of large sclerosing basal cell carcinoma of the nasal dorsum. Subtotal nasal reconstruction with bilateral nasolabial flaps.

10 Facial Reconstruction With Multiple Flaps

Ablative surgery for complex skin cancer and trauma often results in facial defects and deformities that require more than one modality for their reconstruction. In Chapter 8, examples of flaps combined with other modalities were discussed. Upper eyelid tarsoconjunctival flaps were combined with skin grafts for total reconstruction of the lower eyelids. Lateral advancement cheek flaps were combined with nasal cartilage and mucosal composite grafts using the Mustardé technique for similar defects. This chapter will deal with complex defects and deformities requiring more than one flap to effect an adequate reconstruction. Uses of multiple flaps have already been discussed. Chapter 7 covered the Bernard operation, which utilizes bilateral cheek and mucosal flaps for total lower lip reconstruction. When using multiple flaps, it must be remembered that the basic criteria for flap viability and transposition must be met for each involved flap in order to have a successful result.[1] Often when using two flaps, raw flap surfaces are opposed to each other, promoting healing of both. It must also be remembered that when two flaps are used which must later be released, the releasing procedures should be done separately (Figure 76). Some of the multiple flap procedures that have been found to be most useful by the author will be described and illustrated.

MULTIPLE TRANSPOSITION FLAPS

Z-Plasty

The most classic multiple transposition flap technique for facial reconstruction is the Z-plasty. The design of the Z-plasty is that of a Z-shaped figure whose central limb and arms are of equal length. The arms are laid down from each end of the central limb in opposite directions, and parallel to each other so that the two angles thus formed are equal. This technique is often used to lengthen a scar, release a scar tissue band, or change the direction of a scar. The classic angle between the central limb and the arms is 60° but this angle may vary depending upon the amount of lengthening desired. The greater the angle the greater the degree of lengthening. Figure 65 illustrates the use of a Z-plasty to release a post-traumatic contracture of the upper lip and lengthen the scar. This technique is also useful for scar tissue bands and epicanthal folds at the medial canthus (Figure 66).

Multiple Z-Plasty

If a scar to be released or lengthened is long, it is often efficacious to use many transposition flaps in the multiple Z-plasty technique to effect the desired result. If one Z-plasty was used to attempt this in a long scar, large flaps that might widen the area of scarring would be the result. With the multiple Z-plasty technique, the width of the resulting scarring is narrowed and the scar is broken up with more, smaller lines helping to camouflage it. Figure 67 illustrates the use of this method.

Bilateral Nasolabial Flaps

A large nasal skin defect that cannot be closed with a single nasolabial flap may be ideal for the bilateral nasolabial flap technique (see Color Plate I). This may be an excellent alternative when one does not want to use the midline forehead flap for whatever reason, including its thickness.

MULTIPLE INTERPOSITION FLAPS

The most useful multiple interposition flap technique is the geometric broken line closure.[2] This technique evolved from the multiple Z-plasty and the multiple W-plasty.[3] It involves interposing small triangular, rectangular and odd shaped flaps opposed to each other on opposite sides of a scar that is excised. It is a very useful technique in scar excision and scar revision when lengthening of the scar is unnecessary or undesirable. This technique results in a scar that is irregular and therefore less obvious than a straight linear scar, and is very useful in scar revision (Figure 68).

MULTIPLE ROTATION FLAPS

An occasional facial defect will require the use of two rotation flaps in its reconstruction. This technique is most useful in large defects in the area of the temple (Figures 69, 70). When using this technique, the flaps are based anteriorly. The inferior flap is harvested from the cheek while the superior flap is harvested from the temple and forehead. Because of the laxity of the cheek tissues, the inferior flap will rotate considerably further than the superior flap. Both incisions are nicely hidden in the relaxed skin tension lines. The closure line of the two flaps rests horizontally and is often an extension from the lateral canthal area. A standing cutaneous cone has to be excised from the area of joint rotation points of the two flaps.

MULTIPLE FLAPS IN SEQUENCE (SERIAL EXCISION)

Serial excision[4] is a method of excising large benign defects (giant pigmented nevi) or large facial skin grafts with a technique of multiple flaps done in sequence. Large flaps are elevated, usually from the cheek and neck, and stretched so that they are advanced, rotated, or transposed over the abnormality. A significant portion of the abnormality is excised each time. This approach has a great value for large defects which would be impossible to reconstruct in a one stage procedure. This technique is based on the principle of the elasticity of the skin. A three to six month interval is allowed between each procedure. During that period of time, the previously operated skin loosens and another excision is carried out with resulting stretching of the skin once again. It is often remarkable how far the normal skin will stretch in a serial manner such as this.

The patient undergoing these repeated massive flap procedures must be psychologically stable and very well motivated.[5] The patient must understand that Z-plasty, broken line closure, and other scar revisions such as spot dermabrasions may still be necessary to touch up the areas around the new scars and edges of the flaps. Figure 71 illustrates such a complex case, which has required multiple procedures and probably will require more touch-up procedures in the future.

MULTIPLE FLAPS FOR NASAL RECONSTRUCTION

In Chapter 10 we described the midline forehead flap, which is probably the earliest flap to be described for use in facial reconstruction. This is undoubtedly the workhorse flap for major subtotal nasal and midfacial reconstruction. Illustrations of the use of this flap in reconstructing large, deep defects of the medial canthus and nasal ala area have already been presented. A case showing total replacement of the skin of the dorsum of the nose was also shown. In massive tumor resections of the nose, through and through defects are often created. These formidable deformities require an inner mucosal lining replacement as well as external covering and occasionally new structural (cartilage and bone) support. While skin grafts and composite grafts are occasionally useful, secondary flaps in addition to the midline forehead flap are often called for. Several secondary flap techniques to be used in conjunction with a midline forehead flap for full thickness tissue loss will be described and illustrated.

When a large nasal defect also involves a portion of the adjacent cheek or lower eyelid, it is often best to combine a lateral cheek flap with a forehead flap for the reconstruction. This is particularly important when there is an eyelid defect in addition to the forehead defect. Figure 52 showed that the skin of the forehead is a very poor replacement for eyelid skin. The skin of the eyelid is very thin and mobile, while the skin of the forehead is thick and immobile. The texture and even the color match is poor. For this reason it is strongly recommended that forehead flaps not be used in eyelid reconstruction. Figure 72 illustrates a case in which a large lateral nasal defect was combined with a medial lower eyelid defect. This large defect was closed with a combination of a midline forehead flap and a lateral cheek flap. The lateral cheek flap was previously described in Chapter 3. Figure 73 illustrates a large nasal and cheek defect that is closed with a combination of a midline forehead flap and a lateral cheek flap. The forehead flap reconstructs the nasal defect quite nicely, and the tissue of the cheek flap is a much better color and texture match to reconstruct the resultant cheek defect.

When a full thickness nasal defect has been allowed to heal after tumor removal, it is often possible to use turn-in flaps (hinge flaps, flip-flop flaps) to re-create an inner lining and a midline forehead flap for outer lining. Such a case is illustrated in Figure 74. When using turn-in flaps, it must be remembered that the incision cannot be carried down to the edge of the wound or the flap will be devitalized. This technique can also be used on the nasal ala and other areas of the nose. Chapter 2 discussed and illustrated the nasolabial flap for use in external reconstruction of midnasal defects. This flap can be elevated and rotated into the nose with its skin side down to reconstruct an inner lining of a through and through defect, while a midline forehead flap is used to reconstruct the outer lining. This very useful technique is illustrated in Figure 75. The nasolabial flap usually has to be tunneled under adjacent nasal skin and later released. It must be remembered that when two pedicle flaps that are later going to require releasing procedures are used, it is best to stage the releasing procedures.

When a large full thickness ala defect is present that cannot be closed with a fold-over nasolabial flap or a composite graft, a useful technique is the hinged nasal septal flap for inner lining combined with a midline forehead flap for outer lining. This technqiue is illustrated in Figure 76. The septal flap is hinged superiorly. The mucous membrane is removed from the ipsilateral side and left attached to the contralateral side for the inner lining. Cartilage of the septum serves as a nice replacement for the missing lower lateral cartilage. This lends considerable support to the newly reconstructed nasal ala.

DISCUSSION

This chapter has described a variety of multiple flap techniques for the reconstruction of major facial defects. Only the techniques that have been found most useful to the author have been included. The literature is replete with descriptions of other multiple flap techniques that have been found useful by other authors and the reader is referred to other works for more information on this subject.

REFERENCES

1. Conley JJ: Regional Flaps of the Head and Neck. Stuttgart: Georg Thieme Publishers, 1977
2. Webster RC, Davidson TM, Smith RC: Broken line scar revision. Clin Plast Surg 4:263–274, 1977
3. Borges AF: Elective Incisions and Scar Revisions. Boston: Little Brown & Co, 1973
4. Webster RC: Cosmetic concepts in scar camouflaging—serial excision and broken line techniques. Trans Am Acad Ophthalmol Otolaryngol 73:256–265, 1969
5. Cook TA: Use of local skin flaps for scar camouflage. Facial Plast Surg 1:226–239, 1984

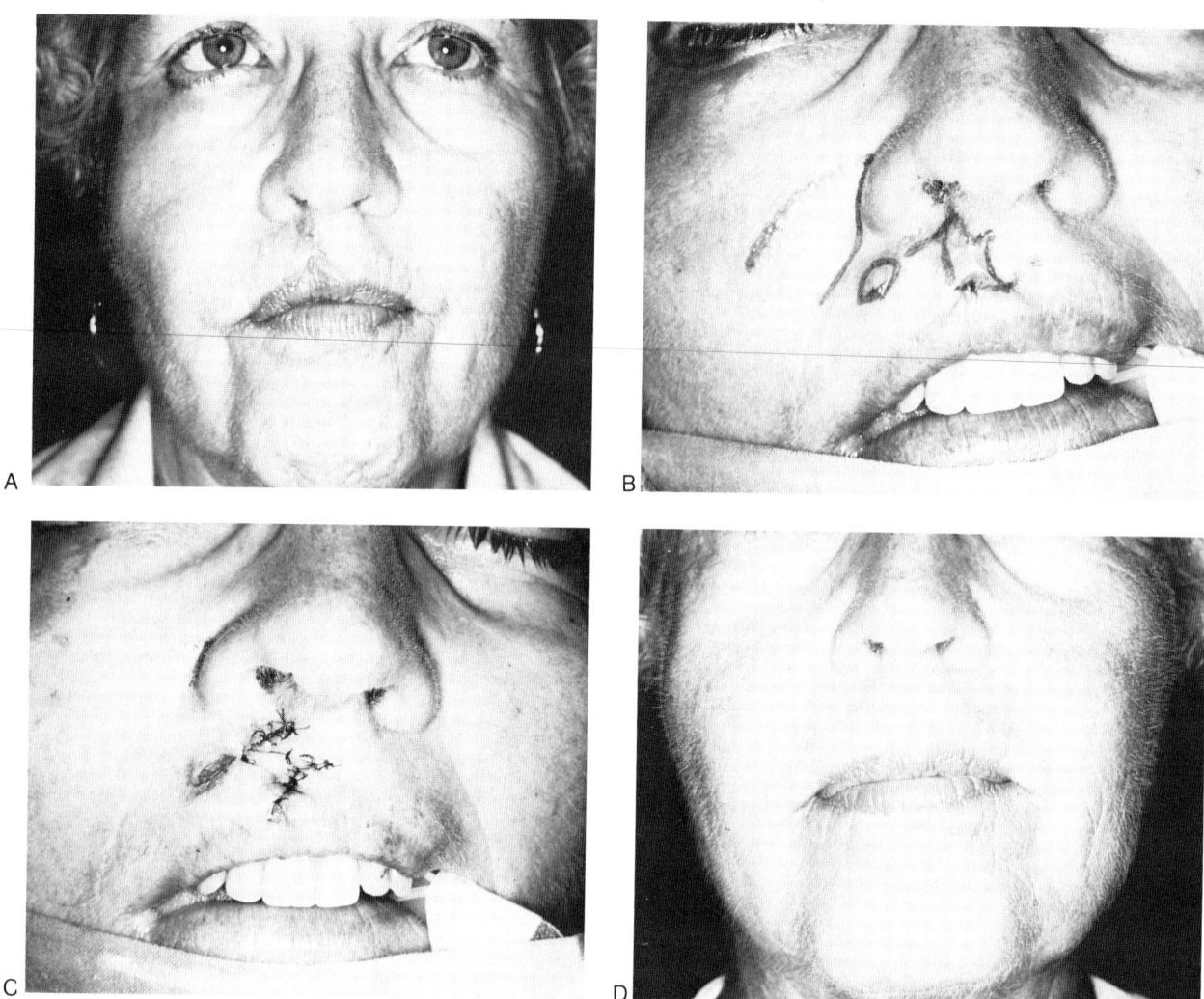

Figure 65. A, Cicatricial contracture of upper lip secondary to previous trauma. B, Scar excision and Z-plasty marked on upper lip. (Disregard other markings.) C, Flaps transposed. D, Final result, one year postoperative.

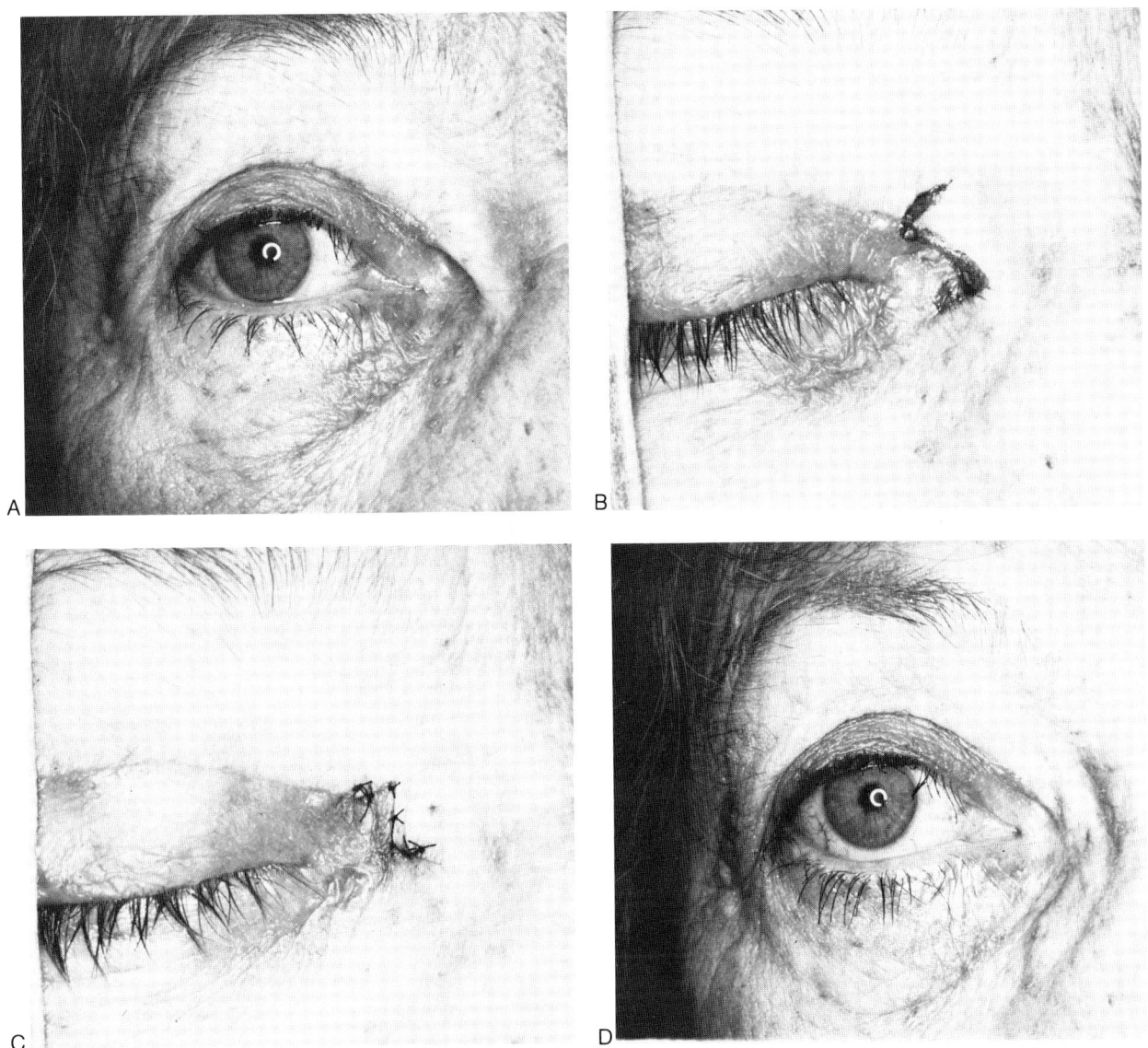

Figure 66. A, Scar tissue band at medial canthus (iatrogenic epicanthal fold). B, Z-plasty marked. C, Flaps transposed. D, Result, four months postoperative.

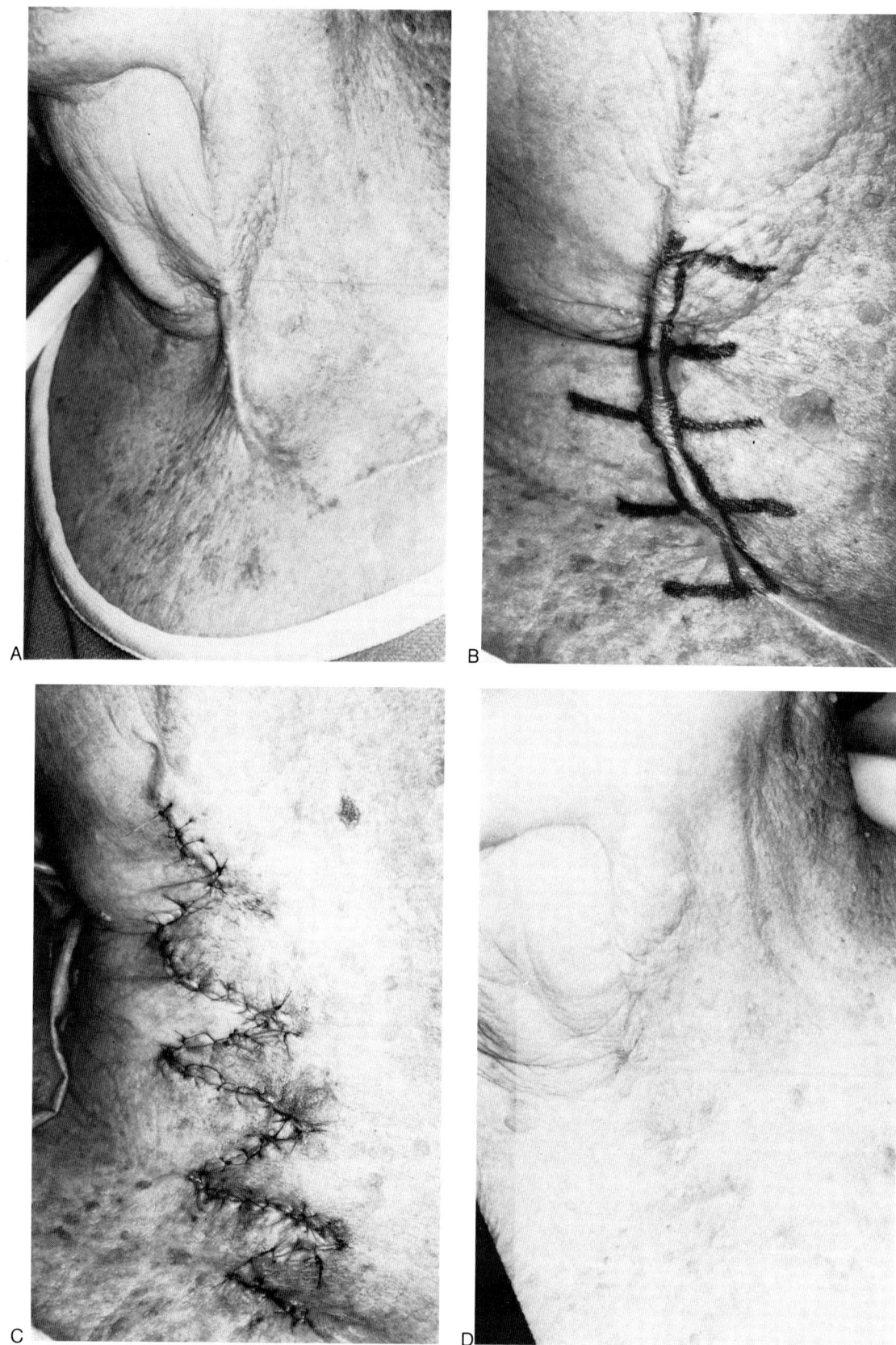

Figure 67. A, Scar tissue contracture of anterior neck. B, Multiple Z-plasties marked. C, Multiple Z-plasty flaps transposed. D, Result, four months postoperative.

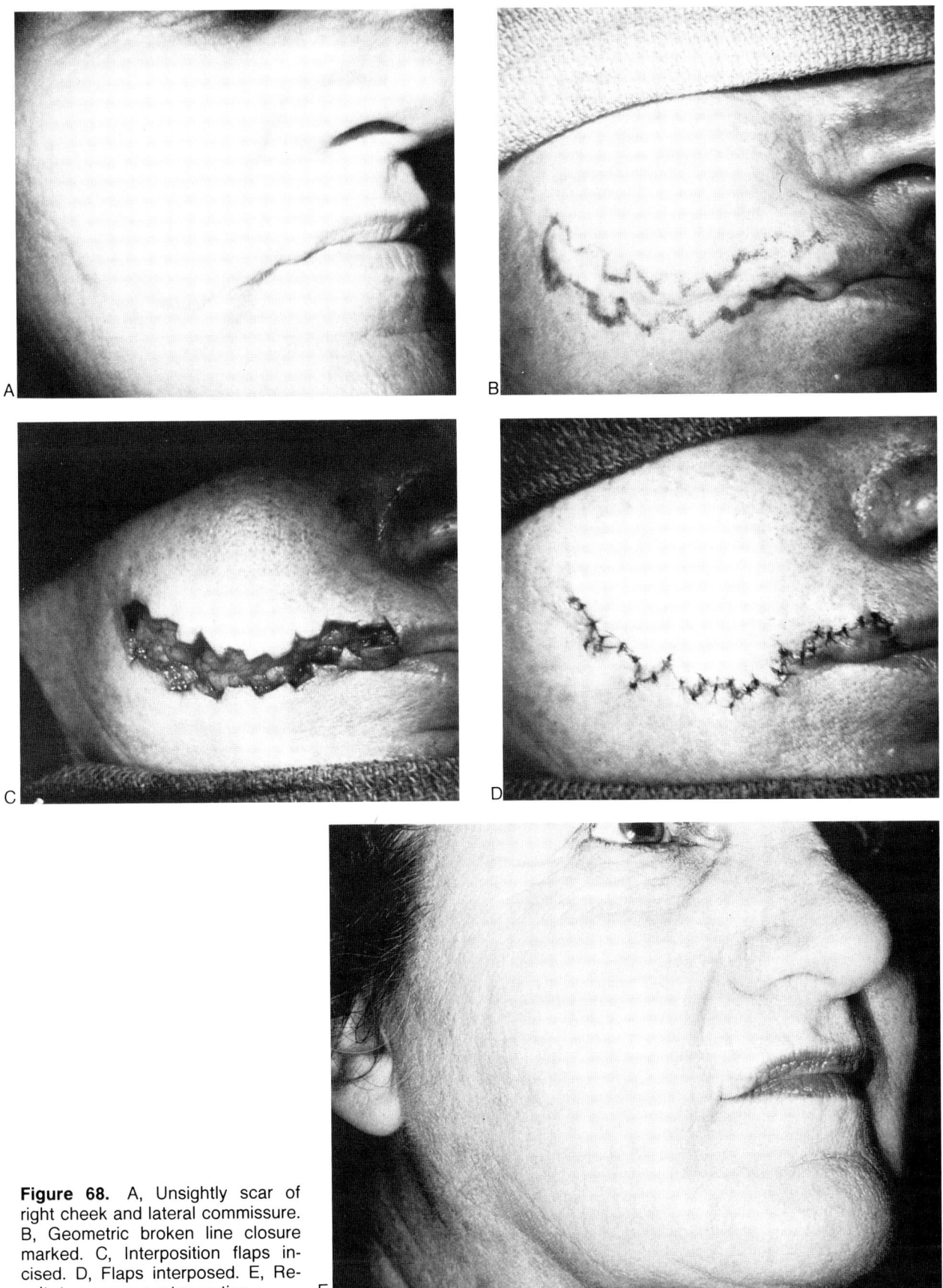

Figure 68. A, Unsightly scar of right cheek and lateral commissure. B, Geometric broken line closure marked. C, Interposition flaps incised. D, Flaps interposed. E, Result, two years postoperative.

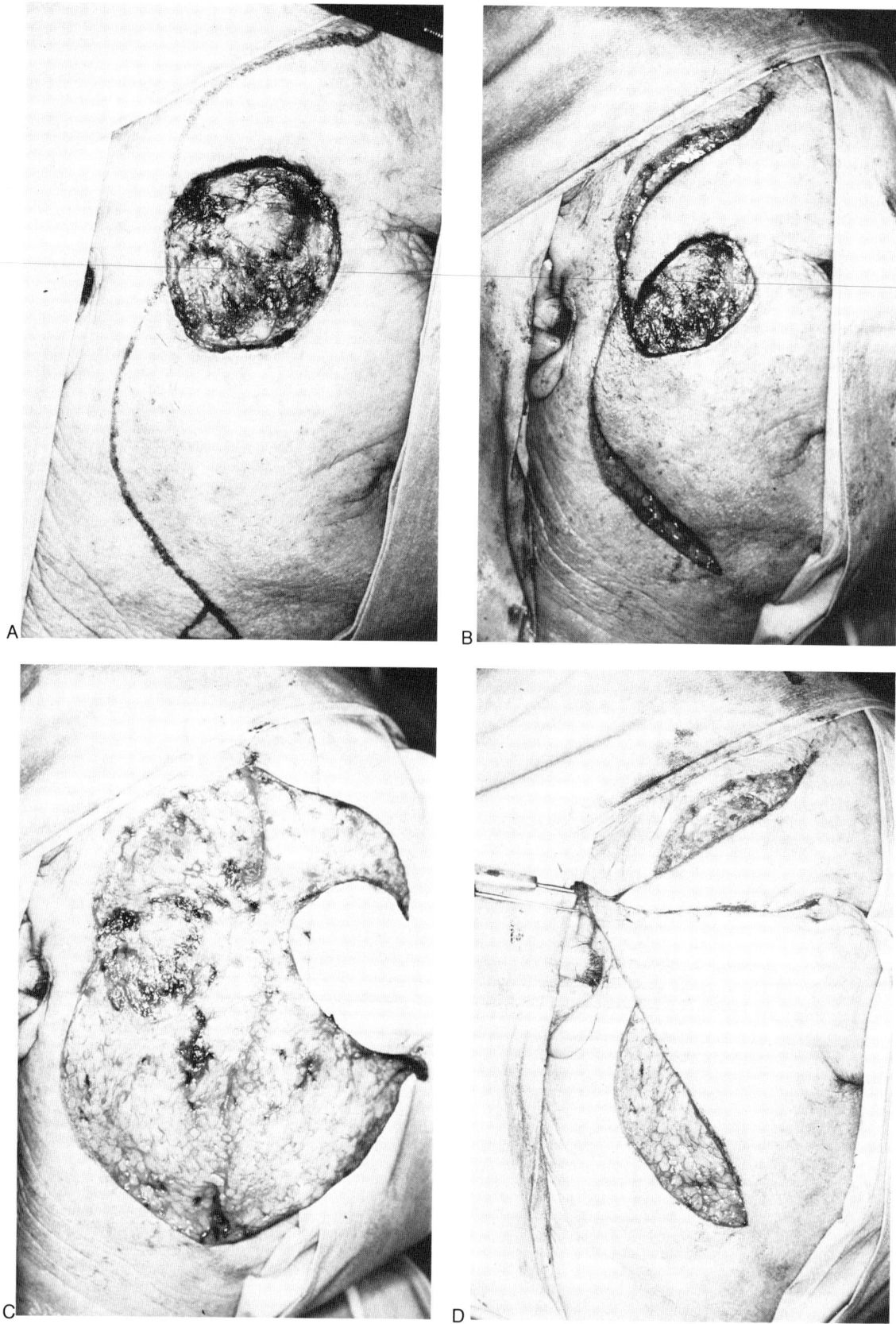

Figure 69. A, Large defect of right temple secondary to excision of recurrent carcinoma by the Mohs' technique. Cheek and temple rotation flaps outlined. B, Flaps incised and undermined. C, Flaps elevated. D, Flaps approximated and excess skin removed.

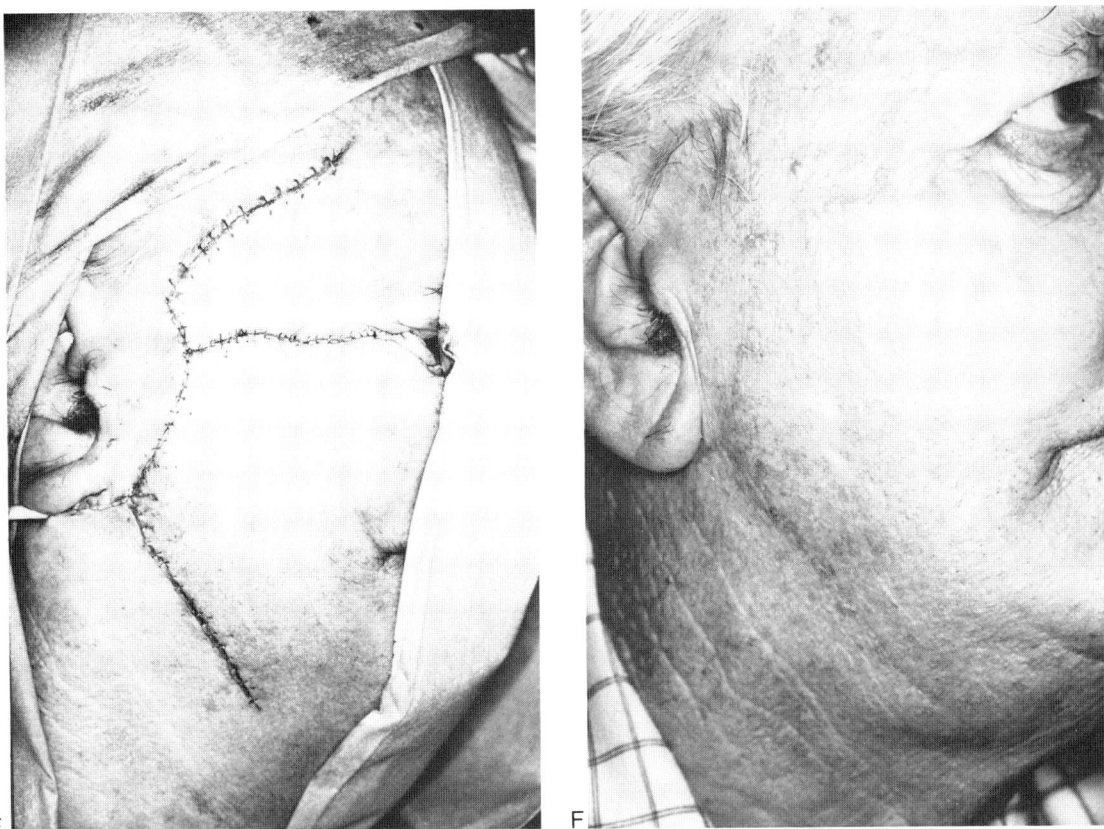

Figure 69 (cont.) E, Final closure. F, Result, four months postoperative.

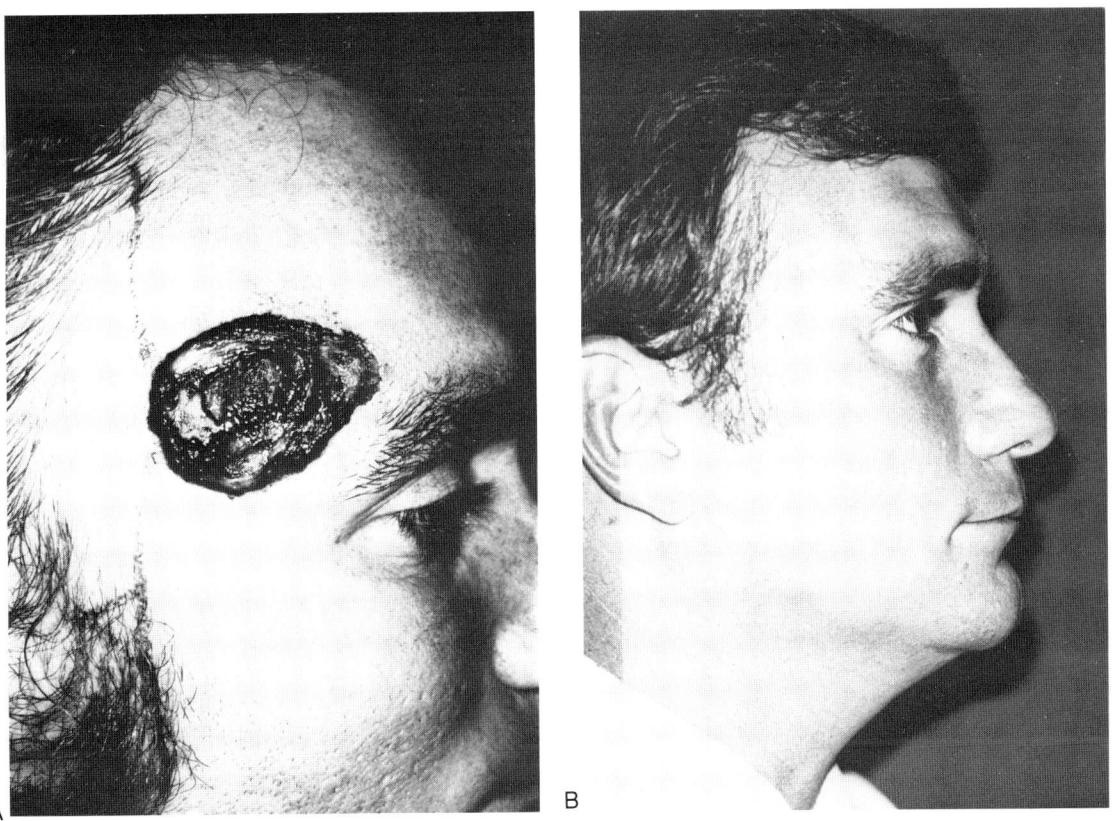

Figure 70. A, Large temple defect secondary to Mohs' excision of recurrent basal cell carcinoma, flaps outlined. B, Result, six months postoperative.

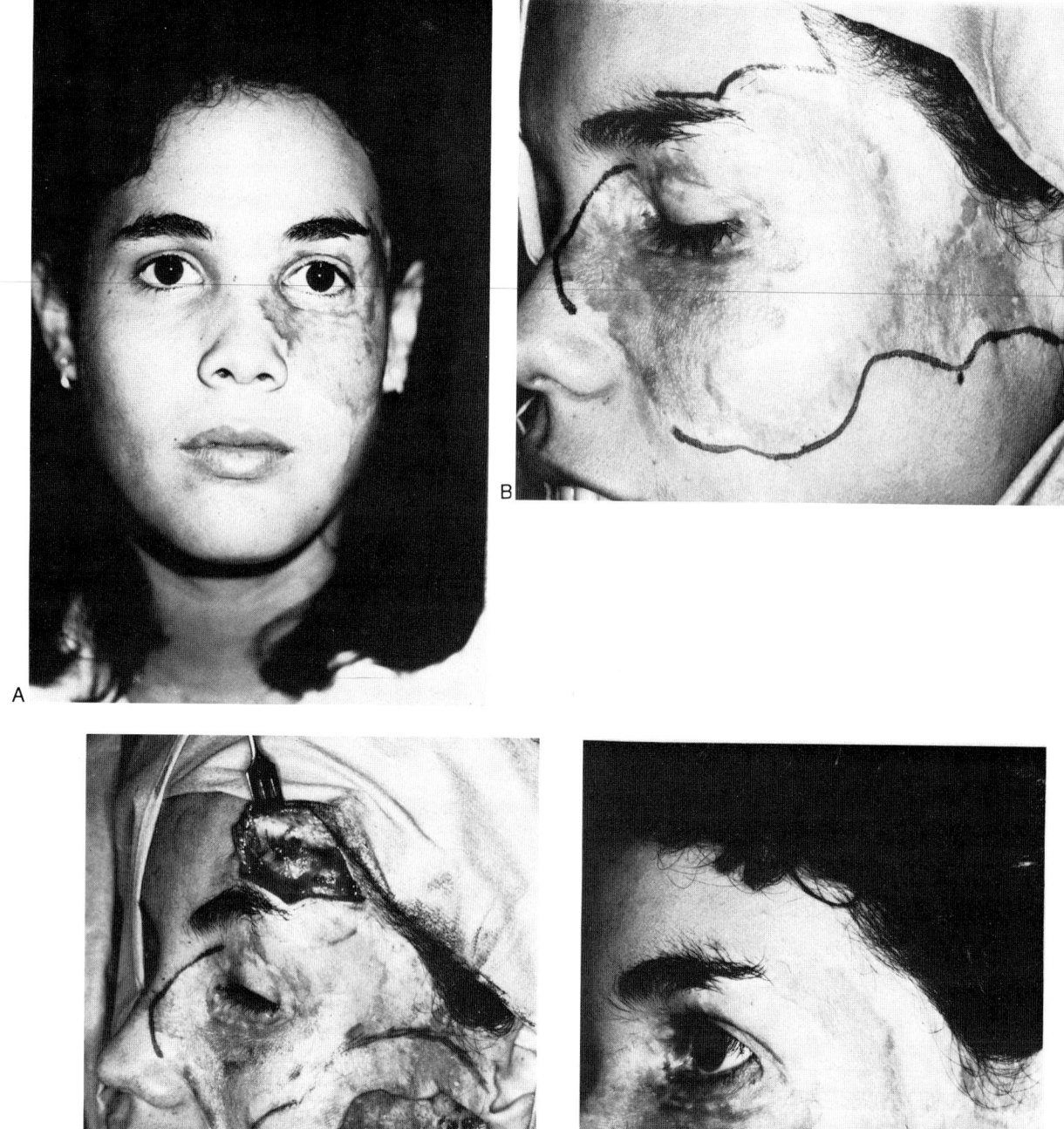

Figure 71. A, 18-year-old female born with giant melanocytic nevus of left face, removed and skin grafted at 9 years of age. B, Outline for first stage of serial excision. C, Flaps elevated, skin marked for proposed excision. D, Postop first stage. Multiple stages were done over a two year period.

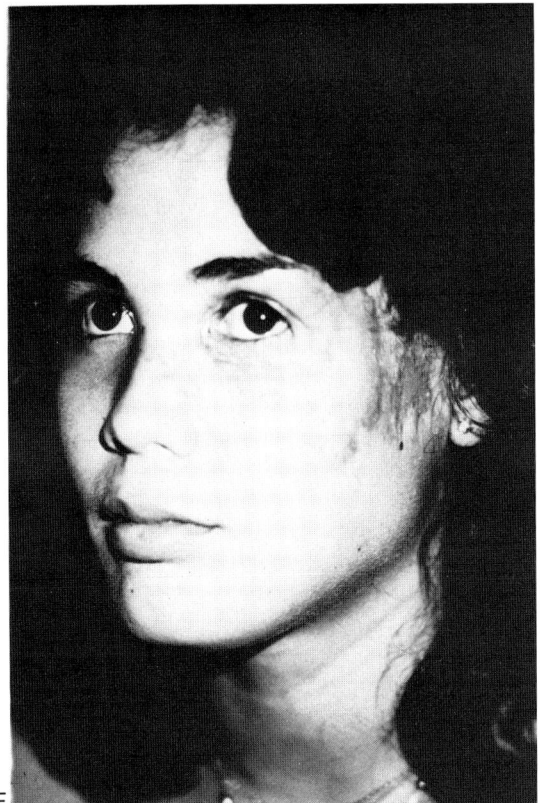 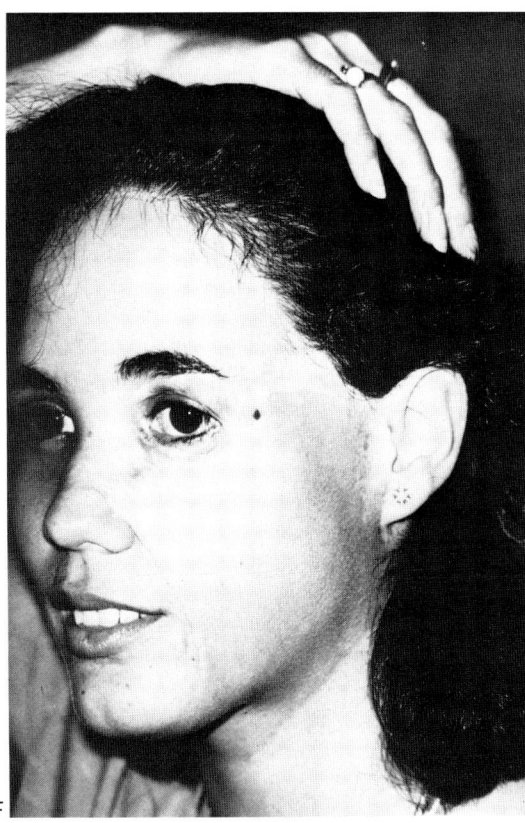

Figure 71. (cont.) E, Preoperative appearance; note small nevus anterior to lobule of ear. F, Six months postop last stage serial excision. Some further revisions will be necessary. Note new position of small nevus which has been preserved lateral to lateral canthus.

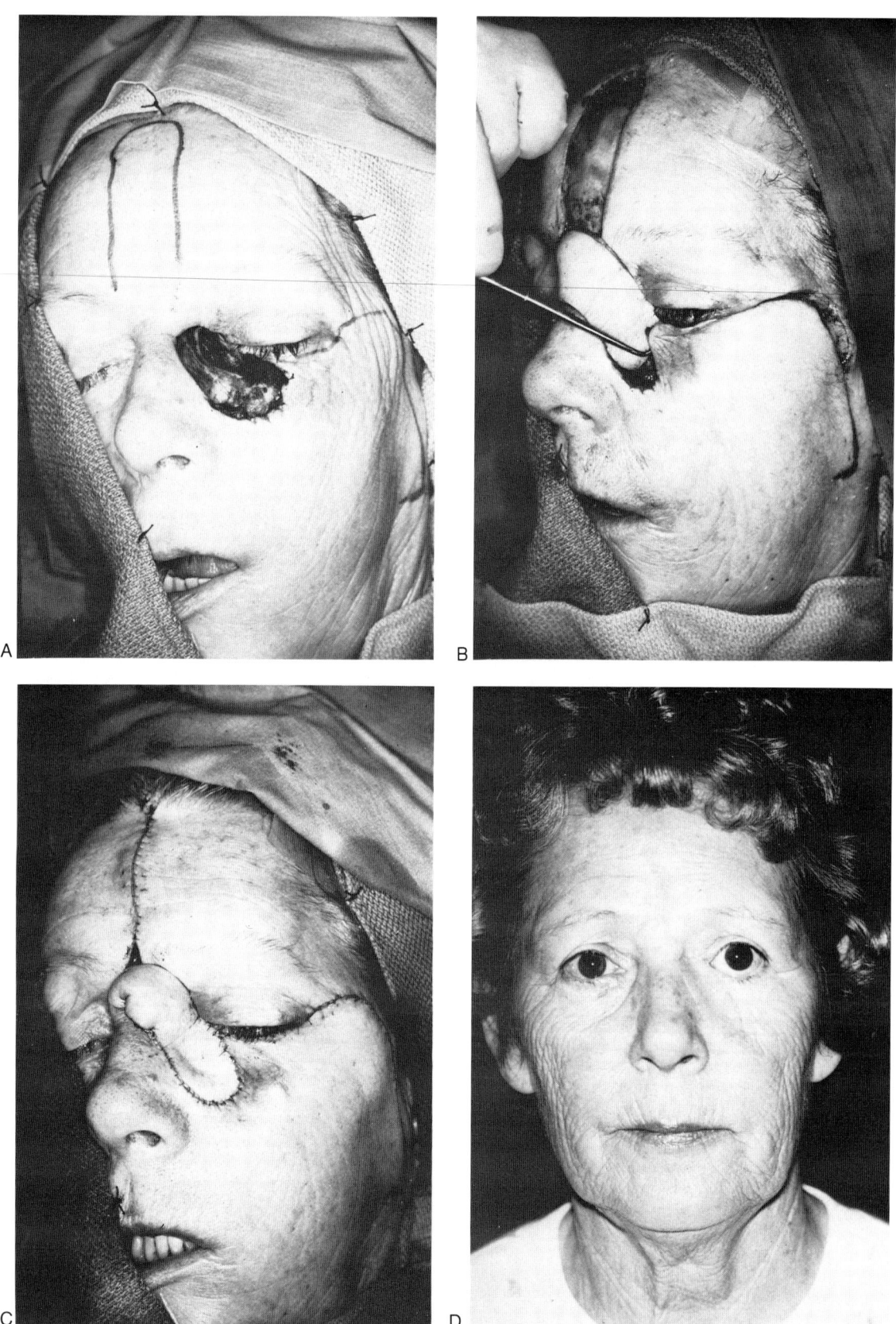

Figure 72. A, Large defect of medial canthus and lower eyelid including lacrimal apparatus secondary to Mohs' excision for recurrent basal cell carcinoma. B, Midline forehead flap and lateral cheek rotation flap elevated and transposed. C, Final closure. D, Result, one year postoperative.

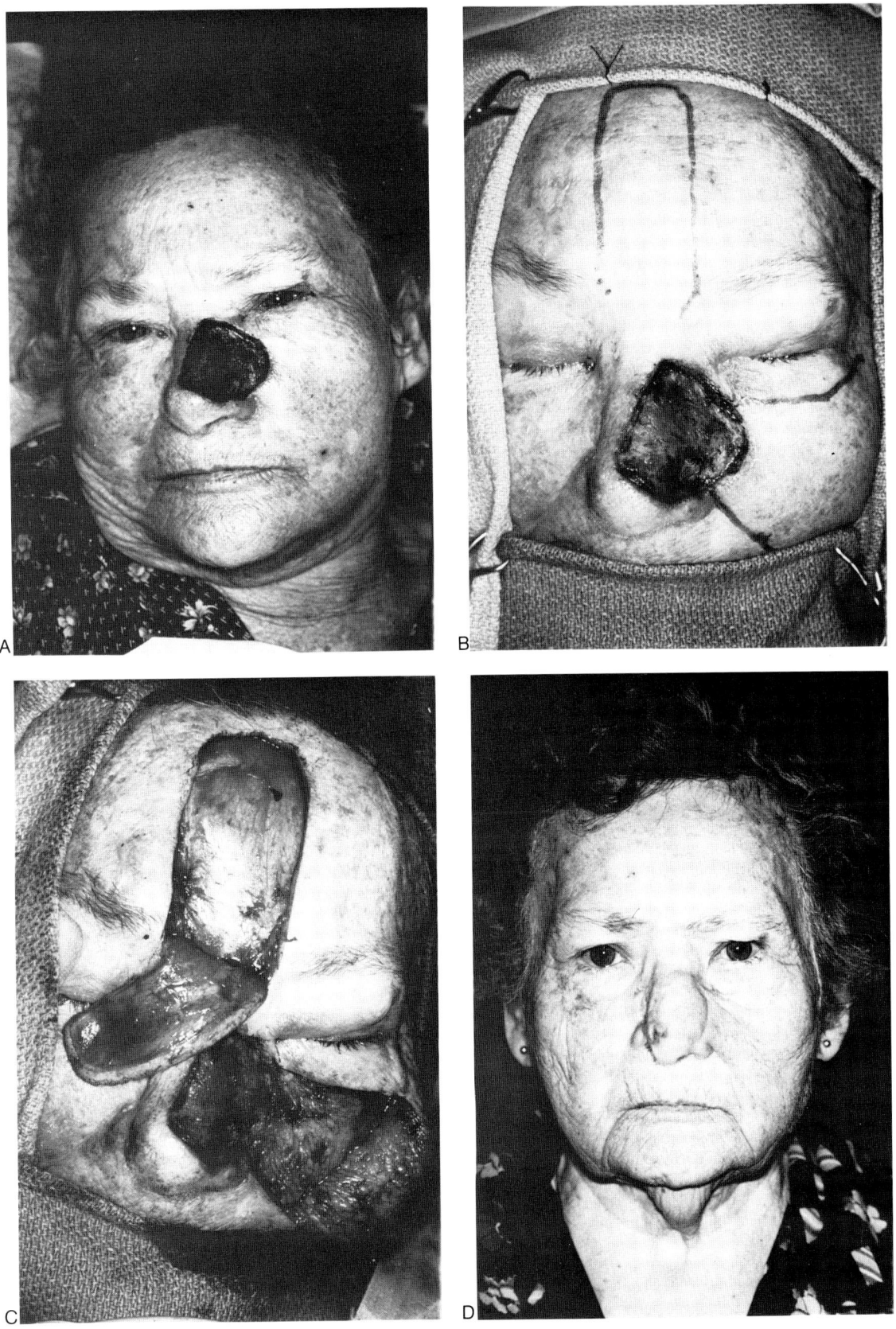

Figure 73. A, Defect following removal of recurrent basal cell carcinoma by Mohs' technique. B, Midline forehead flap and cheek flap outlined. C, Flaps elevated. D, Result, six months postoperative releasing procedure.

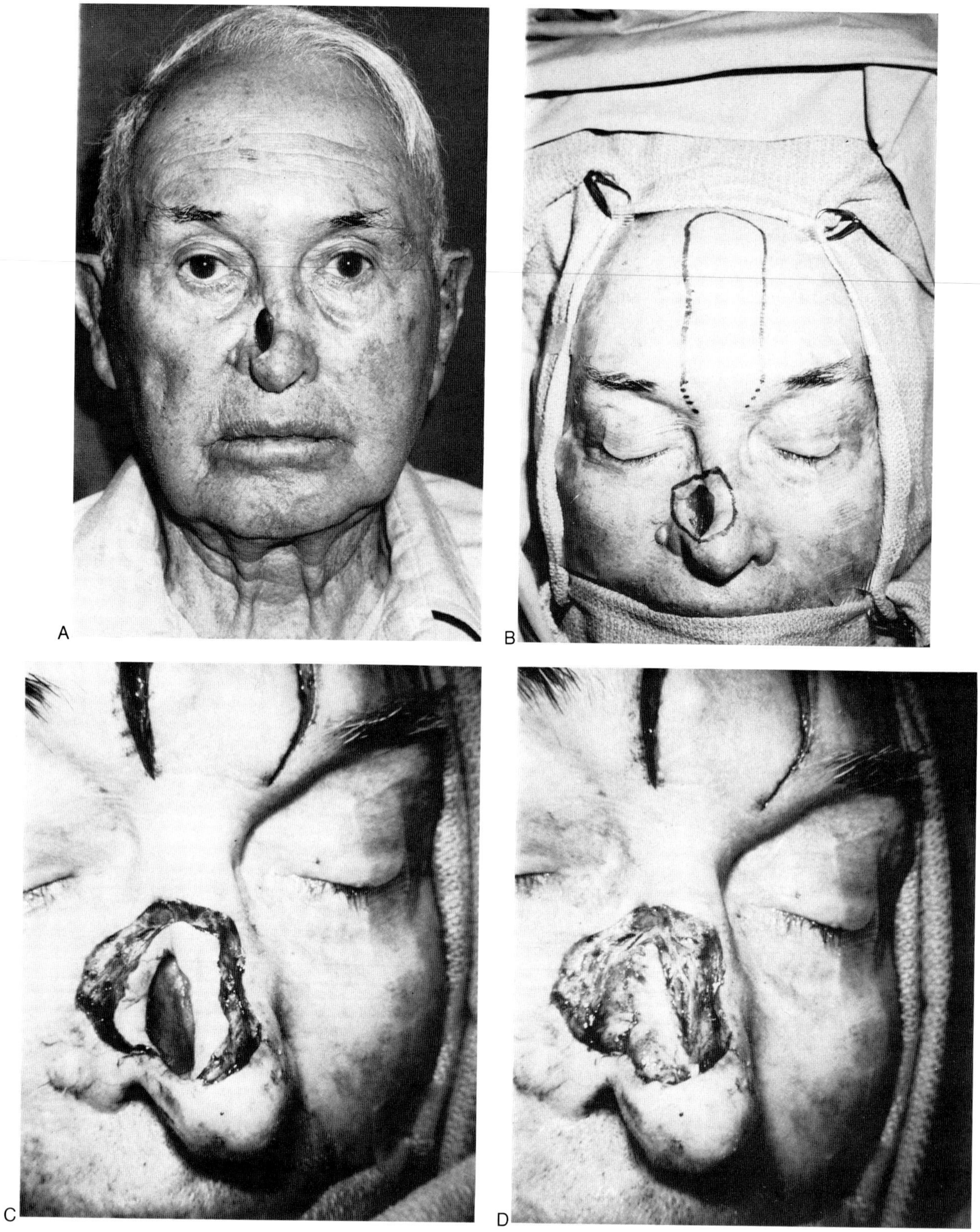

Figure 74. A, Full thickness defect of nose secondary to Mohs' surgery for recurrent basal cell carcinoma, eight months earlier. B, Midline forehead flap and turn-in flaps outlined. C, Turn-in flaps elevated. D, Turn-in flaps sutured together.

Facial Reconstruction With Multiple Flaps 121

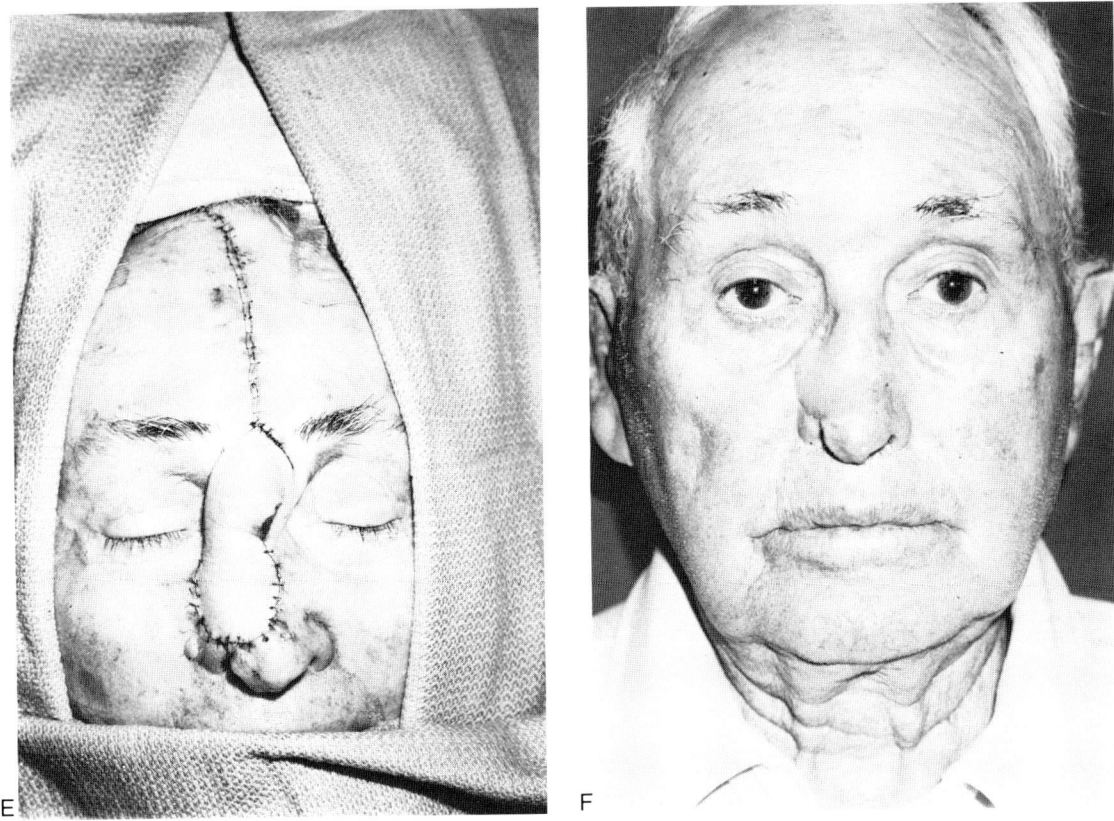

Figure 74. (cont.) E, Final closure. F, Result, one year postoperative.

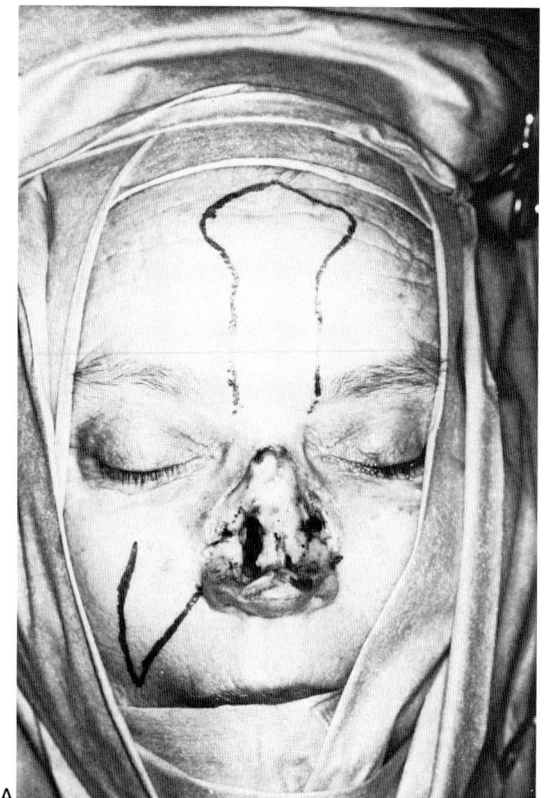
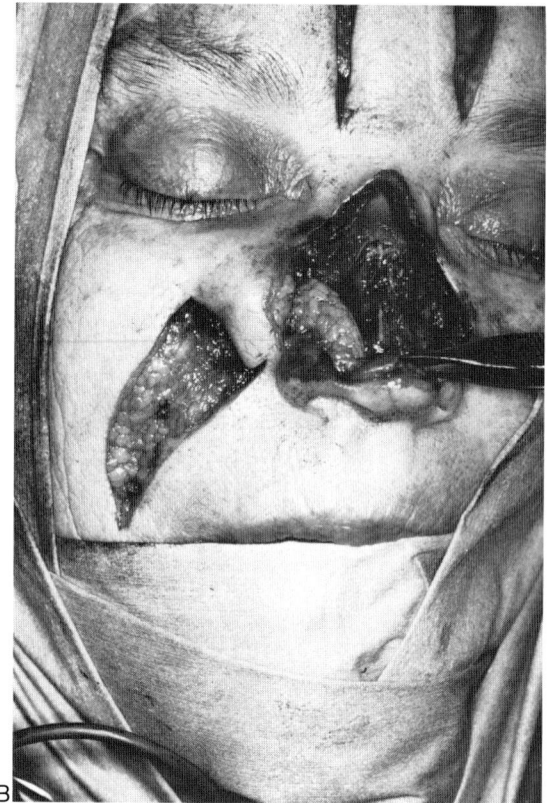
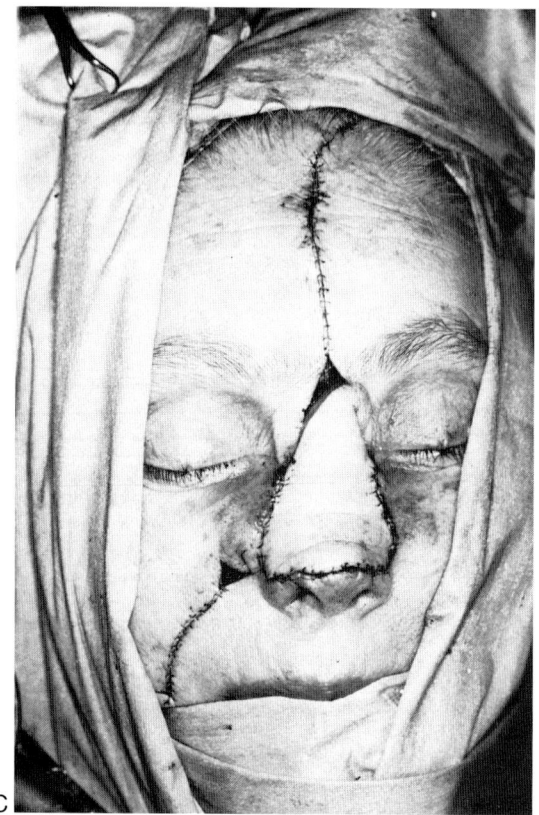

Figure 75. A, Full thickness defect of entire nasal dorsum secondary to previous Mohs' surgery by another physician. Midline forehead flap with extension at distal end outlined for outer covering. Nasolabial flap outlined for inner lining. B, Nasolabial flap tunneled into nose for inner lining. C, Final closure.

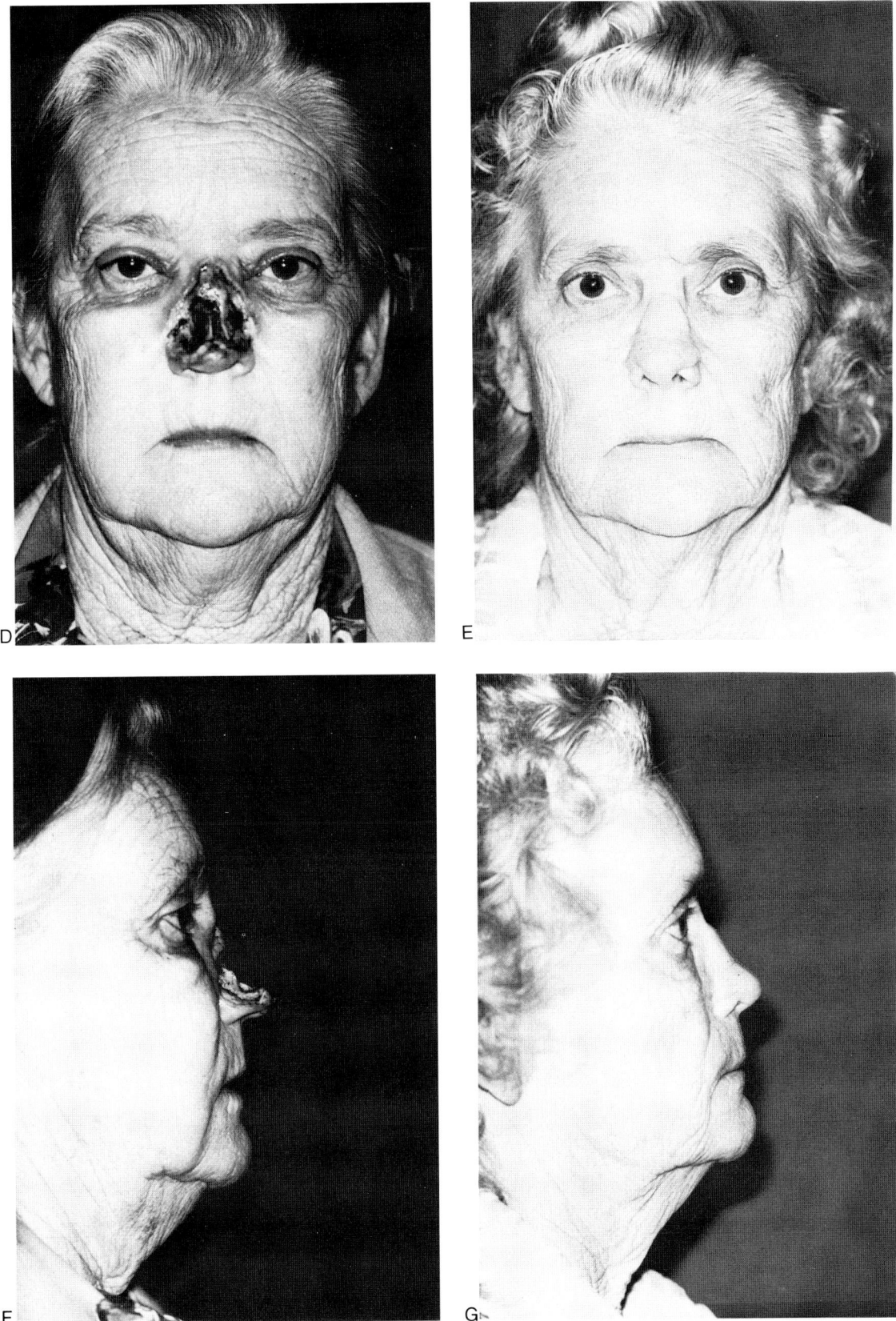

Figure 75. (cont.) D, Frontal view prior to reconstruction. E, Result, four months postoperative release of each flap in stages. F, Lateral view prior to reconstruction. G, Lateral view following reconstruction.

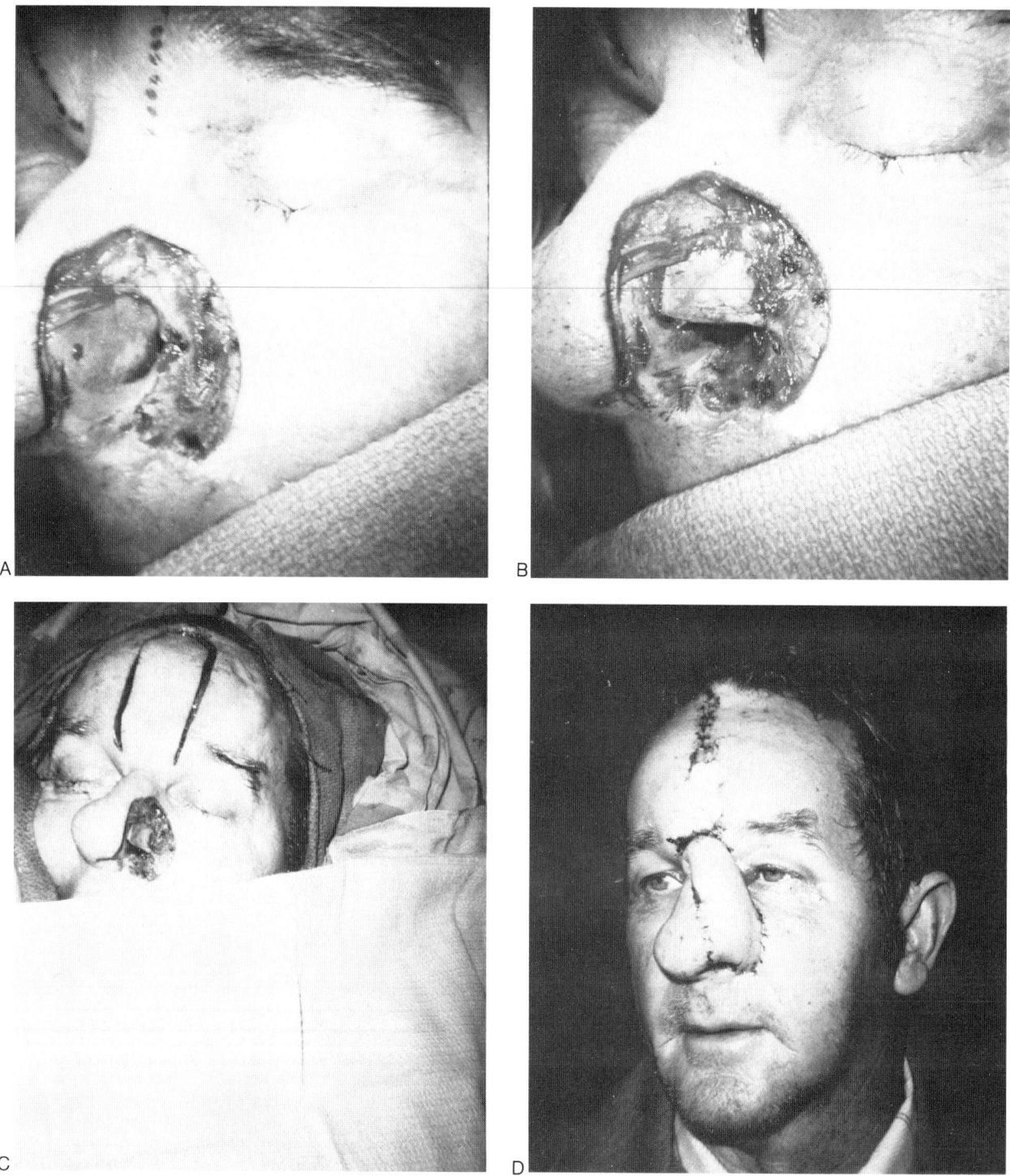

Figure 76. A, Full thickness defect of left nasal ala secondary to Mohs' excision of recurrent basal cell carcinoma. B, Superiorly based hinged nasal septal flap elevated for inner lining, mucosa removed from lateral side. C, Midline forehead flap developed for outer lining. D, Result just before releasing procedure.

Facial Reconstruction With Multiple Flaps 125

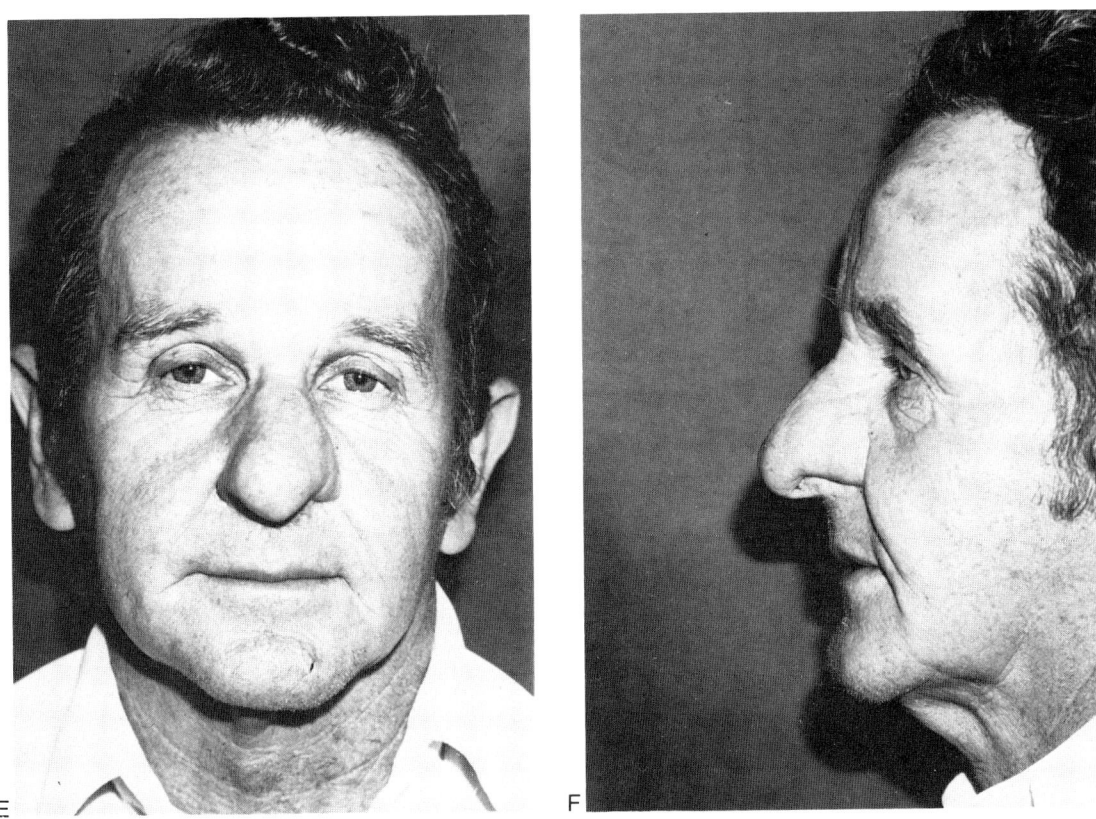

Figure 76 (cont.) E, Final result, one year postoperative, full face. F, Final result, one year postoperative, lateral view.

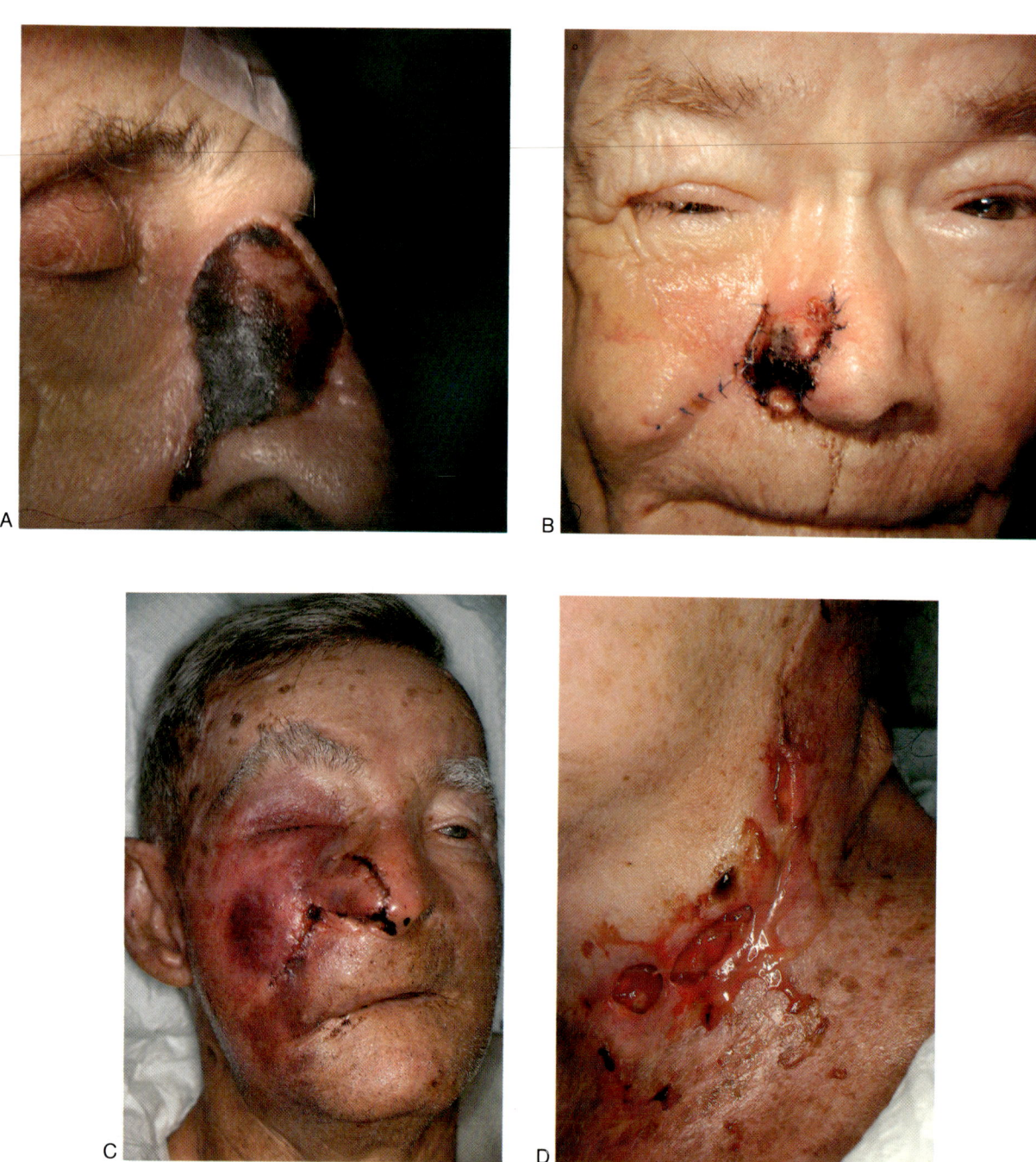

Color Plate II. A. Ischemia, B. Ischemia, C. Hematoma, D. Infection.

11 Complications of Facial Flaps

The possibility that complications might develop is inherent in all human endeavors. This is one of life's greatest truths and one that we are reluctant to accept. Unfortunately, this great truth carries over into surgery. However painful this realization might be for both the surgeon and patient, it must be fully understood by both. Perhaps nowhere are the complications of surgery more apparent and psychologically devastating than in the facial area (Color Plate Two). Conley, in the dedication of his book on the complications of head and neck surgery, spoke of surgical complications by saying: "These untoward events, unpredictable, and unwanted lurk in all surgical arenas, in the biological process and in the patient. They give credence to our frailty, from which there is no escape."[1]

Armed with a clear understanding of these concepts, it behooves facial reconstructive surgeons to study their complications and those of their colleagues in an attempt to predict their possibility and perhaps prevent their occurrence, and to develop a plan for adequately treating them when they do develop. To that end, this chapter will first discuss complications inherent to surgery in general and then move on to those complications that are unique to facial flaps. Prevention and treatment of these unhappy events will be discussed.

In surgery (as in life) there is a tendency to minimize, try to forget about, or otherwise disregard complications. Voluminous literature on the subject of facial flaps has existed for many centuries, particularly in this century. Review of that literature reveals very little discussion on the complications of facial flaps. If the subject is addressed at all it is usually done in less than a page and rarely in several pages. The author hopes that the following will be a meaningful step forward regarding this subject.

COMPLICATIONS INHERENT TO SURGERY

Complications inherent to surgery can be minimized by meticulous adherence to and performance of those known sound principles of good surgical technique, which have been developed by our surgical forebearers. Conley[1] stated it very succinctly when he wrote:

> There are certain *sine qua non*s in surgical technique that can never be taken for granted. Hemostasis should be absolute. All mucous membrane closures should be "spit-tight." Undermining should never be excessive. All flaps should be viable and tissue should not be closed with undue tension. The type and size of the suture material should be appropriate for the job it has to do. Compliance with these fundamental principles establishes the groundwork for healing *per primam* with a minimum of wound complications. When an attempt is made to deviate from these criteria, the incidence of complications will develop in direct proportion to the violation of the principles.

Infection

Fortunately, infection develops quite infrequently (less than 1 percent) in facial reconstructive procedures, and this is considerably less frequently than in general surgical procedures (4 percent). This is probably largely due to the outstanding blood supply that the facial tissues enjoy and perhaps to some degree of regional immunity. When infection does develop in a flap that has just enough blood supply for support, the infection itself may be enough to cause ischemia in a portion of the flap and necrosis in its tip and along the edges of the flap and/or donor site (Figure 77).

The possibility of infection developing can be minimized by the following techniques. The bacterial count on the skin can be markedly decreased by having the patient scrub the face, neck and scalp with an antibacterial soap (Hibiclens) for a few days prior to the surgery. Meticulous aseptic technique in a well equipped, well lighted operating room is vitally important. Recent scientific work on the subject has suggested that the prophylactic use of antibiotics is of dubious value unless a mucosal lined cavity is entered. The author employs antibiotics in major reconstruction of the lips and nose when the mucosal surfaces are involved. Occasionally there will be a delay of one to a few days between the time that a facial skin tumor is extirpated by the microscopically controlled technique of Mohs' and the resulting defect is reconstructed. In these cases antibiotics are used to prevent infection developing in the open wound or in the area of reconstruction. Occasionally antibiotics are used when treating a cancer of the ear involving the cartilage, when there is a significant possibility of perichondritis developing.

Once infection develops, appropriate antibiotic therapy should be instituted immediately, and cultures may be taken to determine the appropriateness of the antibiotic chosen. Any fluctuant areas containing purulent material should be opened and drained promptly. These areas should be allowed to heal by secondary scar tissue contraction. Any resulting deformity secondary to the infection is treated at a later time after it is certain that the infection is completely controlled.

Bleeding

Hemostasis in the surgical wound should be as absolute as is humanly possible. Any significant arterial vessels that are divided should be securely ligated. Electrocoagulation, particularly of the bipolar types, is used vigorously in most wounds. If the recipient and donor wounds are quite large or there is a significant possibility of oozing, drains may be employed. Penrose drains are adequate for smaller wounds and suction evacuation (Hemovac) is used for very large wounds. Light pressure dressings are often applied and may be helpful. Great care should be employed in the use of pressure dressings in facial flap procedures to avoid compression of the vascular supply of the flap.

If a significant hematoma develops (probably about 4 percent of major facial procedures), the wound should be opened, the hematoma evacuated, and the bleeding vessels coagulated. Following this the wound is closed and redressed. Small hematomas that are not expanding or compromising the vascular supply of the flap may be managed by watchful waiting (Figure 78). A large expanding hematoma that is not evacuated can cause compromise to the vascular supply of the flap with subsequent slough and loss of skin. This possibility should be avoided at all costs.

Injury to Normal Uninvolved Structures

A thorough knowledge of the anatomy of the face and neck is vital prior to undertaking any facial reconstructive or flap procedure. Knowledge of the facial blood supply is necessary to plan a well vascularized flap properly and to prevent injury to the feeding vessels. It is important not to injure any major adjacent vessel which might be needed for another flap or reconstruction at a future time. An understanding of the cartilaginous and bony framework of the nose and face is needed to prevent unnecessary injury to these structures during tumor removal and reconstruction. Occasionally it is necessary to remove some normal cartilage and bone in reconstructing a nose to decrease the bulk of the flap reconstruction and to give a more normal postoperative aesthetic appearance. Adjacent cartilage (Figure 76) or bone is sometimes used in the reconstructive process with a facial flap.

Nerves are the main uninvolved structures which can be inadvertently or purposely sacrificed in a facial flap reconstructive procedure, causing the most disfigurement. Figures 78 and 80 are illustrative cases where the frontal (temporal) branch of the facial nerve was inadvertently severed. Damage to the marginal branch of the facial nerve is a possible occurrence when the operation is carried deep to the platysma muscle in the lower face and below the lower border of the mandible. Conley, Baker and Selfe[2] recently reported on the biology of this abnormality and an excellent method to correct it (Figure 81). The main trunk and the two major divisions of the facial nerve are located within the parotid gland deep to the lobule of the ear and are rarely injured in facial flap procedures, unless a parotidecetomy is carried out in conjunction. Even then, injury to the facial nerve itself is rare in competent hands. The most vulnerable sensory nerve in the face is the supraorbital nerve. This nerve is at risk in deep dissections of the medial brows and medial forehead areas. The infraorbital and mental nerves are deeply located and rarely injured.

Failure to Control Tumor

Recurrent skin cancer under and around a flap reconstructive procedure because of inadequate control of the original tumor is perhaps the worse complication of facial flaps. This complication is probably worse than losing a flap entirely. If a flap is lost, the area can be debrided and another procedure performed. If recurrent tumor is discovered in and under a flap, not only does the entire flap have to be removed but a large surrounding cuff of diseased tissue as well as some undiseased tissue has to be removed to clear the area of tumor. Microscopic evaluation of all malignant skin tumors removed should be carried out for diagnosis and completeness of tumor removal. There are certain instances where more exacting techniques are required. Fredric Mohs[3] developed a technique for the microscopically controlled excision of skin cancer, which bears his name. Microscopically controlled excision (Mohs) is strongly recommended for skin cancers that are recurrent following previous attempts at removal or radiation therapy. The technique is considered essential in morphea-type (sclerosing) basal cell carcinomas, which have clinically inapparent margins and are often much larger than anticipated (Figure 82). Menn and co-workers[4] compared the cure rates of conventional surgery with Mohs' surgery for recurrent basal cell carcinoma. They found that the cure rate for conventional surgery in recurrent basal cell carcinoma was only 50 percent while that for Mohs' surgery was 96 percent. The Mohs' technique not only has the advantage of a considerably higher cure rate for these difficult tumors, but has the additional advantage of conservation of more normal tissue than standard surgical techniques. Only the tissue that has been traced out microscopically to contain tumor and a small cuff of noninvolved tissue need be removed. Therefore as much normal tissue as possible is preserved. For this reason, the microscopically controlled technique of Mohs' is particularly useful for tumors of the eyelids, nose and ears. In these areas the anatomy is more complex, tumors tend to be more extensively involved, and there is less excess tissue with which to reconstruct than in the cheeks and other areas of the face. A good rule of thumb is not to plan a facial flap reconstructive procedure unless the chances of cure of the underlying facial skin cancer is exceptionally high. Figure 83 demonstrates a case in which a nasolabial flap was used to reconstruct a defect created by the excision of skin cancer only to have recurrent cancer develop in the suture line a year or more later. The extent of excision necessary to render a tumor free plane is also demonstrated and is impressive.

Biological Problems of the Patient

The possibility of underlying medical problems should be explored prior to performing an operation. So it is with patients on whom a facial flap is contemplated. There are certain medical conditions which are known to predispose a patient to complications in this type of surgery. These have been broken down into the following classifications.

Systemic Diseases

Diabetes, arteriosclerosis, and hypertension are all well known for their effect on the blood vessels of the arterial side of the circulation. These diseases can decrease the blood supply to flaps. Diabetics are considerably more prone to infection than patients without this disease. Hypertension not only can cause vascular spasm, but it also increases the possibility of other complications such as hematoma formation. These diseases should be under medical supervision and as controlled as possible prior to undertaking surgery.

Immunologic Diseases

Patients with compromised immunologic systems and those on immunosuppressive therapy often exhibit delayed wound healing and can have significant complications when flap surgery is performed (Figure 84). A consultation with the patient's internist, immunologist, or oncologist is helpful in treating these patients.

Hematologic Diseases

If the patient has a history of a bleeding tendency, this problem should be evaluated. The author routinely employs a prothrombin time and partial thromboplastin time in addition to complete blood count in evaluating patients for major facial surgery. It is important to question patients regarding aspirin therapy and antiarthritic medications which are known to cause prolonged bleeding. Patients are asked to stay off of all aspirin containing products for at least two weeks prior to surgery.

Radiation Induced Problems

Patients who have had previous radiation therapy have increased scar tissue and decreased blood supply to the irradiated tissues. There is less tendency for primary healing in these patients. This problem should be appreciated by the surgeon and the patient prior to surgery. A flap from an adjacent or regional non-irradiated area can often bring in fresh viable tissue to reconstruct the area successfully.

Skin Diseases

Contact dermatitis, psoriasis and other skin disorders can interfere with healing of the skin and should be as controlled as possible prior to surgery. The effects of aging on the skin can cause increased capillary fragility and bruising as well as atrophic changes to the skin such as thinning of the epidermis and dermis.

Self-Induced Problems in Patients

A specific history should be sought regarding the amount of alcohol consumption and smoking. Heavy consumption of alcohol will dilate blood vessels and predispose the patient to the development of bleeding and hematoma. In addition, alcoholics have a high rate of cirrhosis and decreased liver function causing bleeding and other healing problems. It has become recognized in recent years that heavy smoking is associated with a significant increase in the possibility of skin loss in flap procedures. Patients who are having major facial surgery are asked to abstain from smoking at least two weeks prior to surgery. Compliance with requests to decrease drinking and smoking is unfortunately quite low.

COMPLICATIONS UNIQUE TO FLAPS

There are certain complications that are unique to flap surgery. These problems will be discussed and illustrated.

Problems of Blood Supply

As mentioned in the first chapter on classification, all local and regional flaps can be divided on the basis of their blood supply into random pattern flaps and axial pattern flaps. Random pattern flaps have their blood supply based on the subdermal plexus, while axial pattern flaps depend on a direct named cutaneous artery for their primary blood supply. While it is obvious that the plan to the flap should include an adequate blood supply, it should be equally obvious that every effort should be made to maintain the integrity of the vascular system to the flap. To that end, all dissection under random pattern flaps should be in the subcutaneous plane and should not violate the subdermal plexus, which is located just below and sometimes attached to the undersurface of the dermis. Great care should be taken when dissecting the pedicle of an axial pattern flap to prevent injury to its feeding vessel or vessels.

Loss of blood supply with subsequent ischemia is the most feared complication of flap procedures. Figure 85 demonstrates the loss of a portion of the tip of a random pattern transposition flap that appeared to be well designed and executed. It can only be assumed that some damage occurred to the underlying subdermal plexus in this case. Figure 86 illustrates a case in which the base of the flap was designed in an area of previous scarring. This probably resulted in loss of the distal end of the flap. Figure 87 demonstrates the total loss of an axial pattern flap. When these untoward events occur, the area of ischemia is allowed to demarcate. Devitalized tissue is debrided as indicated over a period of time. Remarkably, in most of these cases the bed in which the flap was placed often will heal by secondary scar tissue contraction with surprisingly good results.

Lymphedema and Thickening

When a flap is planned, incised and raised, the lymphatic and smaller vascular channels are cut to at least three sides of the skin that is utilized in the flap. As a result, it is not uncommon for facial flaps to have persistent edema as previously shown in Figures 15 and 52. Often this lymphedema and thickening will decrease over several months subsequent to the flap procedure. It is difficult to tell which flaps will exhibit this problem. It has tended to be more common in nasolabial and forehead flaps than in most others, in the author's experience. When the problem occurs and does not correct itself with time, debulking (defatting) procedures (Figure 88) are recommended. These procedures are usually carried out through one or two of the previous incisions, and the edges of the scars are revised at the same time. Occasionally, an incision will be made in the direction of a natural skin fold such as the nasal crease if this has partially been obliterated by the flap. The skin is elevated under not more than half of the flap surface. The underlying thickened tissues are then removed enough to allow the flap to lay back in a more normal configuration. One or two of these procedures is usually adequate but occasionally several are required. Bennett[5] suggested that virtually all patients undergoing nasal reconstruction with skin flaps require at least one revision and often as many as three. In the author's experience, secondary procedures to debulk or revise flaps are necessary in considerably less than half of all nasal reconstructions.

Mechanical Factors

It cannot be overemphasized that as a facial flap is incised and raised, every effort must be exerted to protect the flap and its blood supply. To that end, it is strongly suggested that the flap not be stretched. Stretching of a flap may avulse or tear the small vessels of the subdermal plexus and cause problems of ischemia. Stretching in the form of significant tension at the edge of the wound, particularly at the corner of the flap, can cause partial loss (Figure 89). Gravity can be a significant problem with downward pull on the flap. Chapter 3 discussed the importance of anchoring a cheek flap that is used to reconstruct the lower eyelid at the lateral canthal area of the orbital rim with an anchoring suture from the dermis to the periosteum of the rim. When this anchoring has not been done properly or even despite the best efforts of the surgeon, some pull-down or ectropion can be the result (Figure 90). Twisting or bending may be a problem (Figure 87) and undue compression on the base of the flap can result in tissue loss (Figure 91).

Problems of Planning and Design

For most flaps to be successful, every effort should be made to plan and design facial flaps to meet the criteria that have been well established. Earlier chapters of this book have included those criteria outlined over the years by innovators and leaders in this field. Donor site scars and as many of the flap scars as possible should be planned to fall in natural skin folds in the lines of relaxed skin tension. Efforts should be made not to distort normal anatomical landmarks as was emphasized in the chapter on rhombic flaps. One must think of where the rotation point of the flap will be and the possibility of a resulting standing cutaneous cone (dog ear). Adequate tissue should be designed in the flap to cover the defect. Mechanical factors such as gravity and twisting should be considered. Flaps should be planned that will be appropriate for the reconstruction to be undertaken. Figures 92 though 96 illustrate five flap procedures that had flaws in their planning and design phase, resulting in less than optimal results.

DISCUSSION

Complications will inevitably develop in some facial flap procedures despite the best planning, design and execution of the procedure by the surgeon. This chapter has been an attempt to discuss and illustrate the complications of facial flap surgery that might be encountered. Particular emphasis has been placed on measures designed to decrease the possibility of complications with additional emphasis on the successful treatment of complications when these unwanted events occur. It is hoped that this discussion will encourage other surgeons who operate in the facial area to analyze the complications of their flap procedures and those of their colleagues, to increase our knowledge on this subject further. This endeavor might help countless patients in future years.

REFERENCES

1. Conley JJ (ed): Complications of Head and Neck Surgery. Philadelphia London Toronto: WB Saunders Co, 1979
2. Conley JJ, Baker DC, Selfe RN: Paralysis of the mandibular branch of the facial nerve. Plast Recon Surg 70:569–676, 1982
3. Mohs FE: Chemosurgery for skin cancer. Arch Dermatol 112:211–215, 1976
4. Menn H, Robins P, Kopf AW, Bart RS: The recurrent basal cell epithelioma. Arch Dermatol 103:628–631, 1971
5. Bennett JE: Reconstruction of lateral nasal defects. Clin Plast Surg 8:587–598, 1981

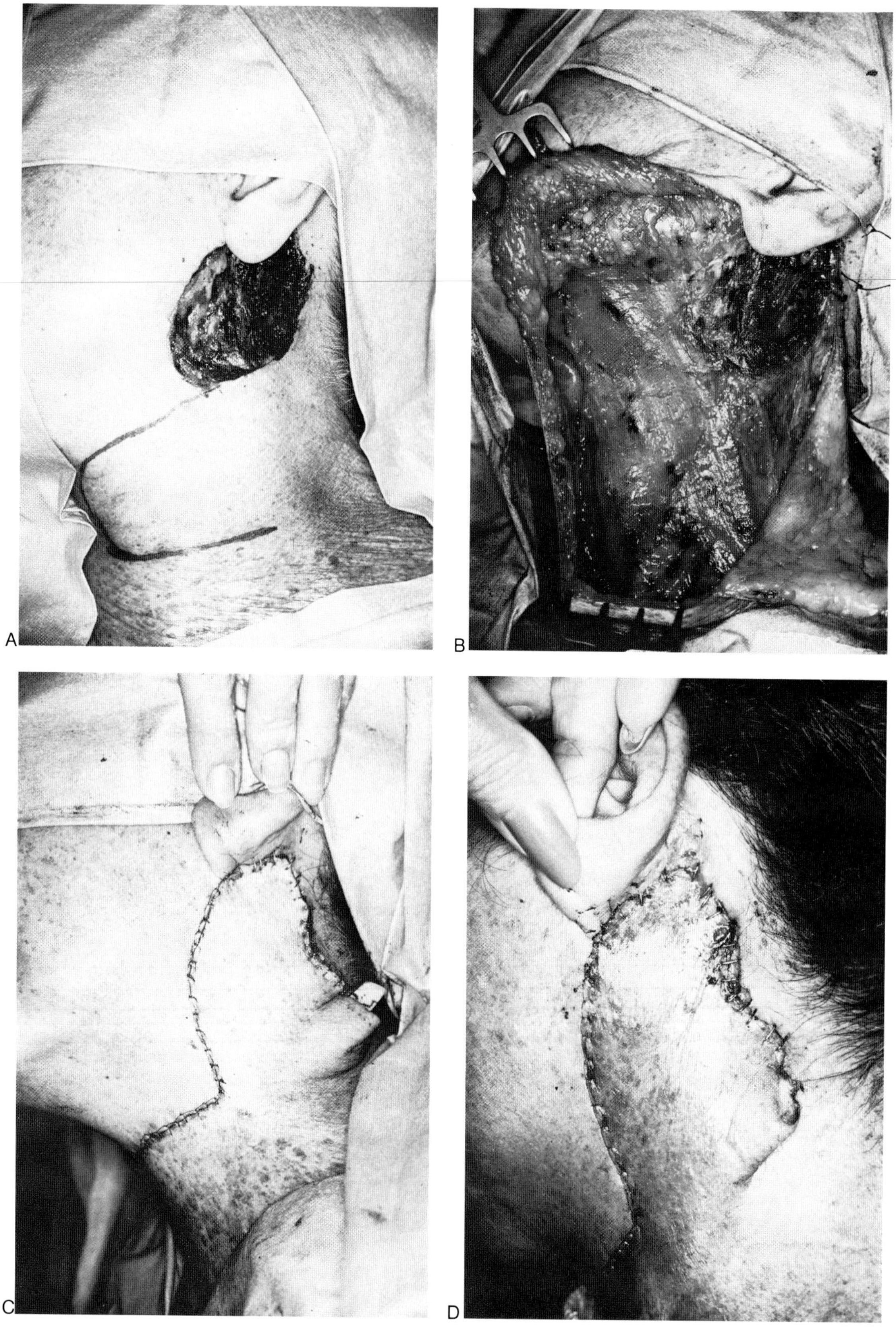

132 Facial Reconstruction with Local and Regional Flaps

Figure 77. A, Defect resulting from excision of recurrent basal cell carcinoma by Mohs' technique; horizontal neck flap outlined. B, Flap elevated in plane just superficial to platysmal layer. C, Final closure, standing cone left to avoid interruption of blood supply of flap. Later removal was planned. D, Five days postoperative, infection under flap with ischemia of distal segment.

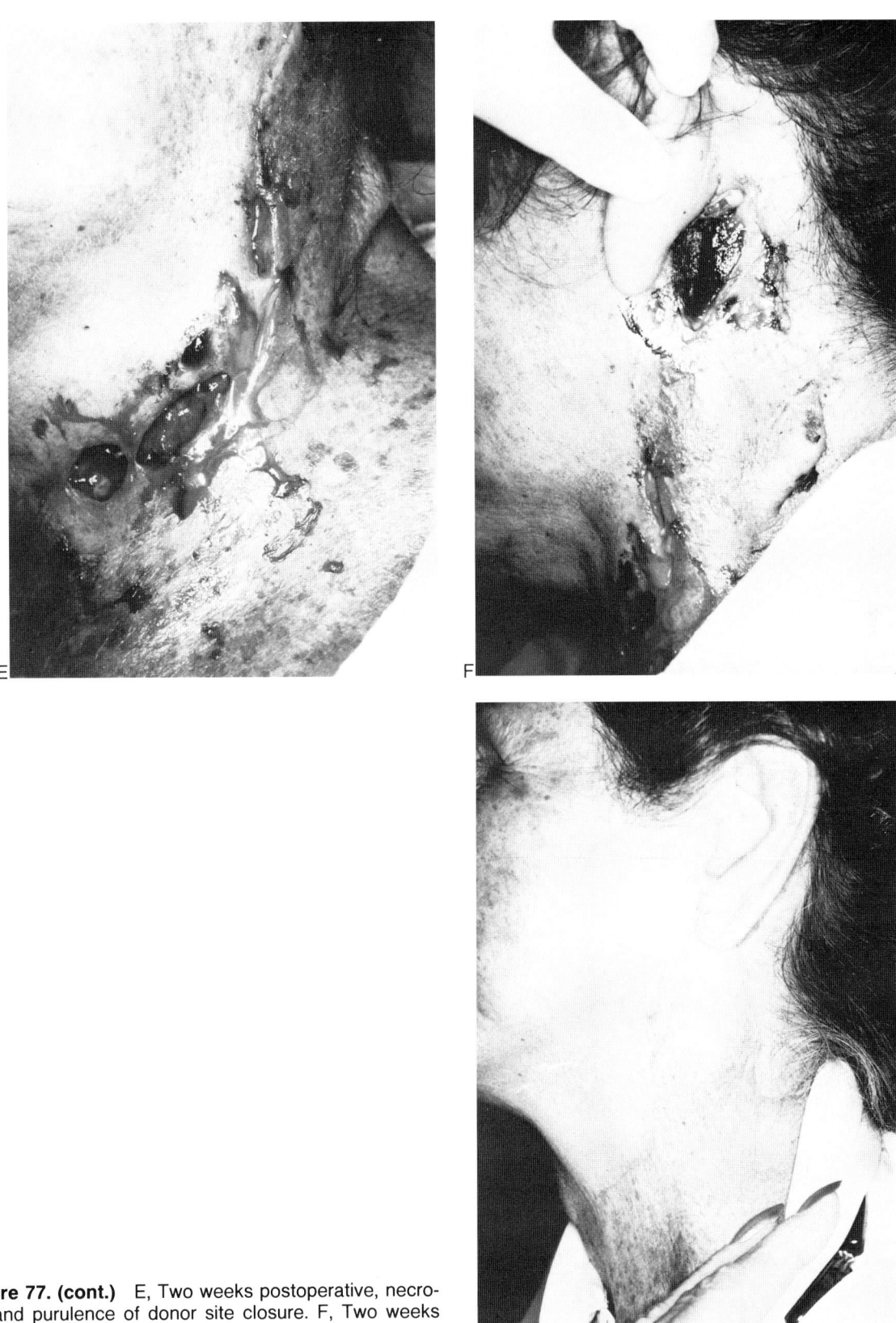

Figure 77. (cont.) E, Two weeks postoperative, necrosis and purulence of donor site closure. F, Two weeks postoperative, necrosis of tip of flap. G, Final result, one year postoperative, spontaneous healing.

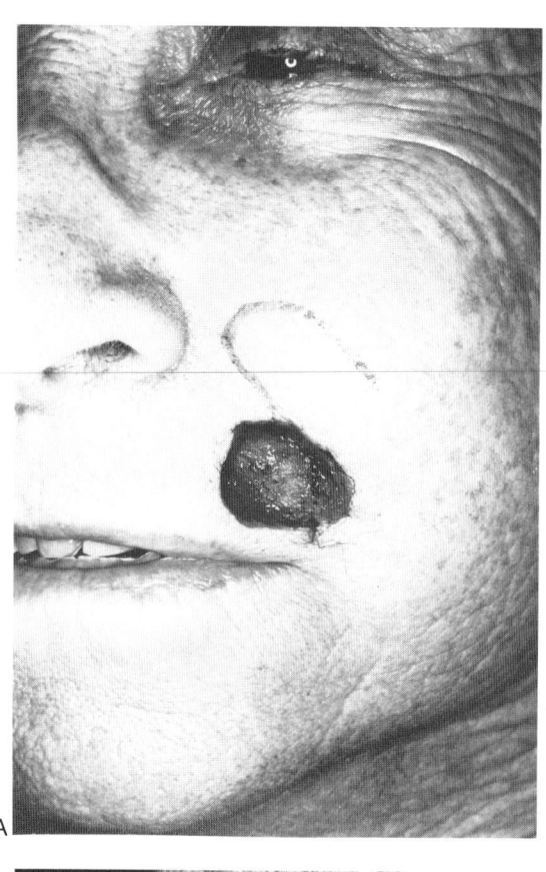
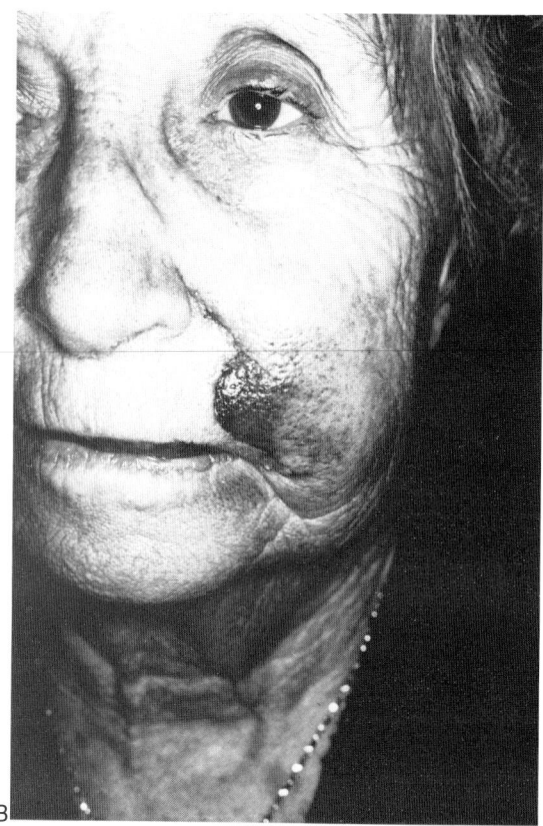
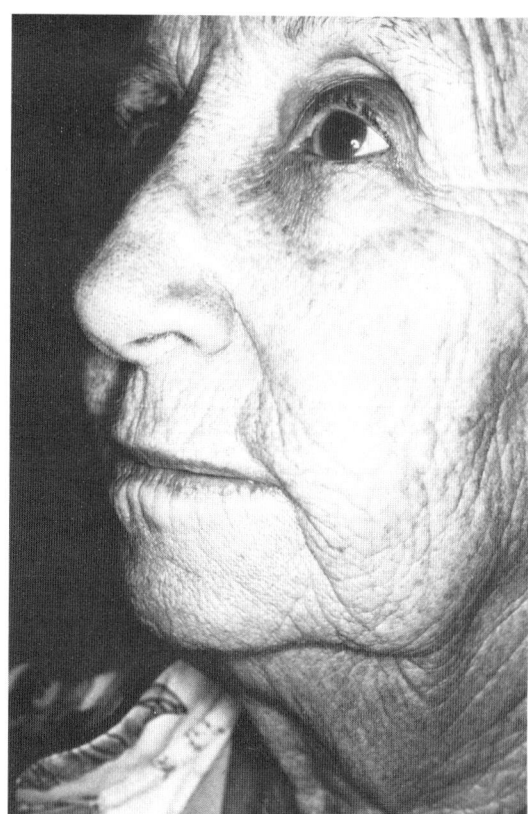

Figure 78. A, Nasolabial flap planned for upper lip defect. B, Moderate hematoma developed, not requiring drainage. C, Final appearance, four months postoperative.

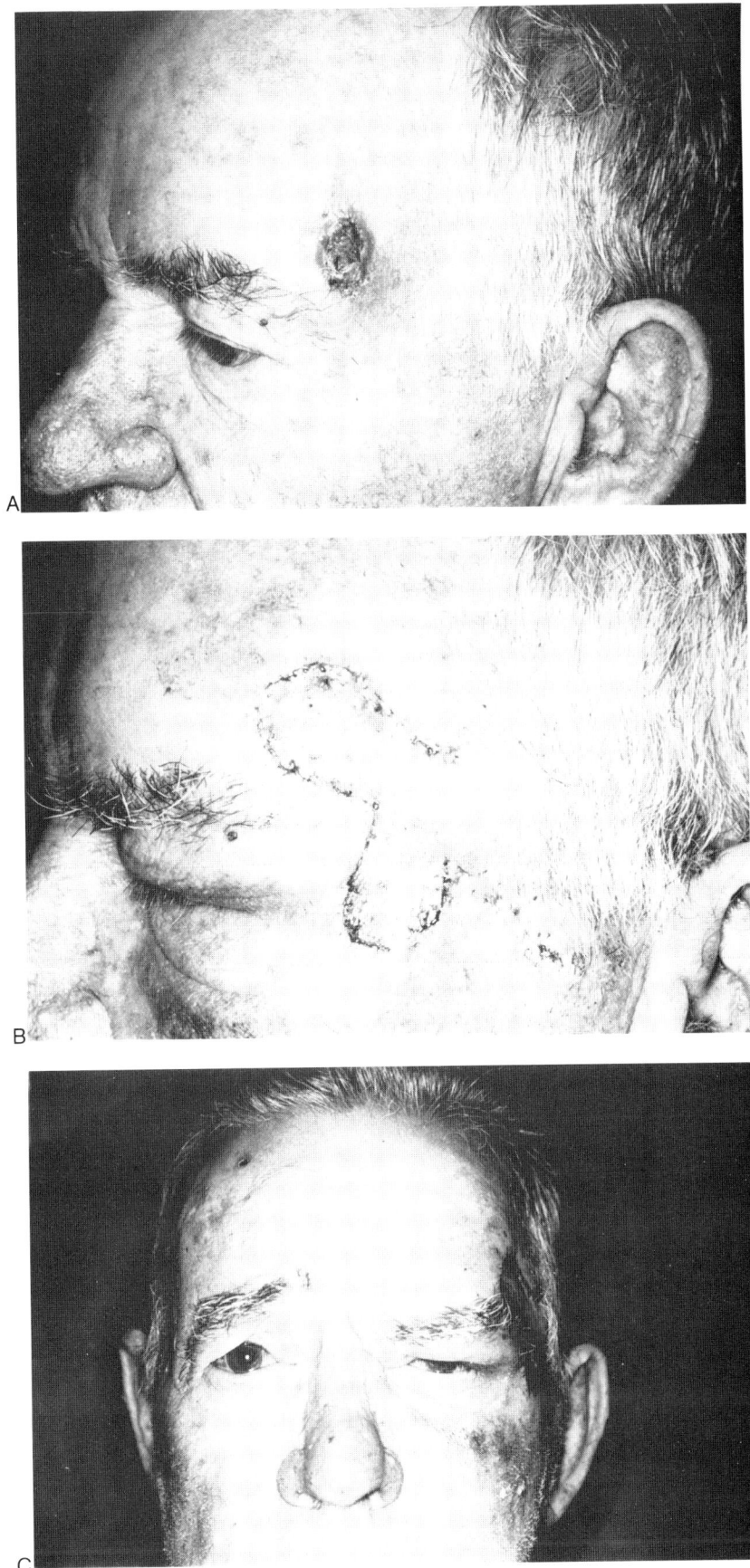

Figure 79. A, Large basal cell carcinoma of left temple, directly over temporal branch of facial nerve. B, Immediate postoperative status; bilobed flap by another surgeon. C, Paralysis of temporal branch of facial nerve on left side with significant brow ptosis.

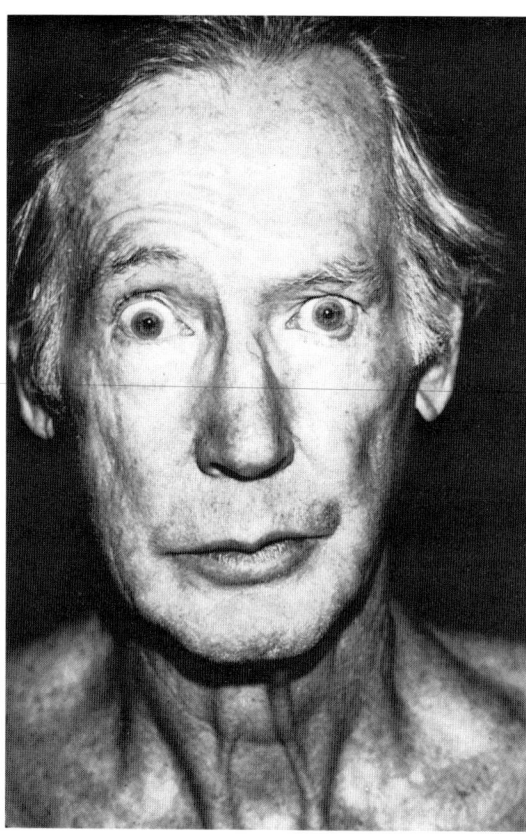

Figure 80. The patient had a left lower eyelid reconstruction with the Mustardé technique by another plastic surgeon several years prior to this photograph. Note paralysis of left forehead on raising of brows.

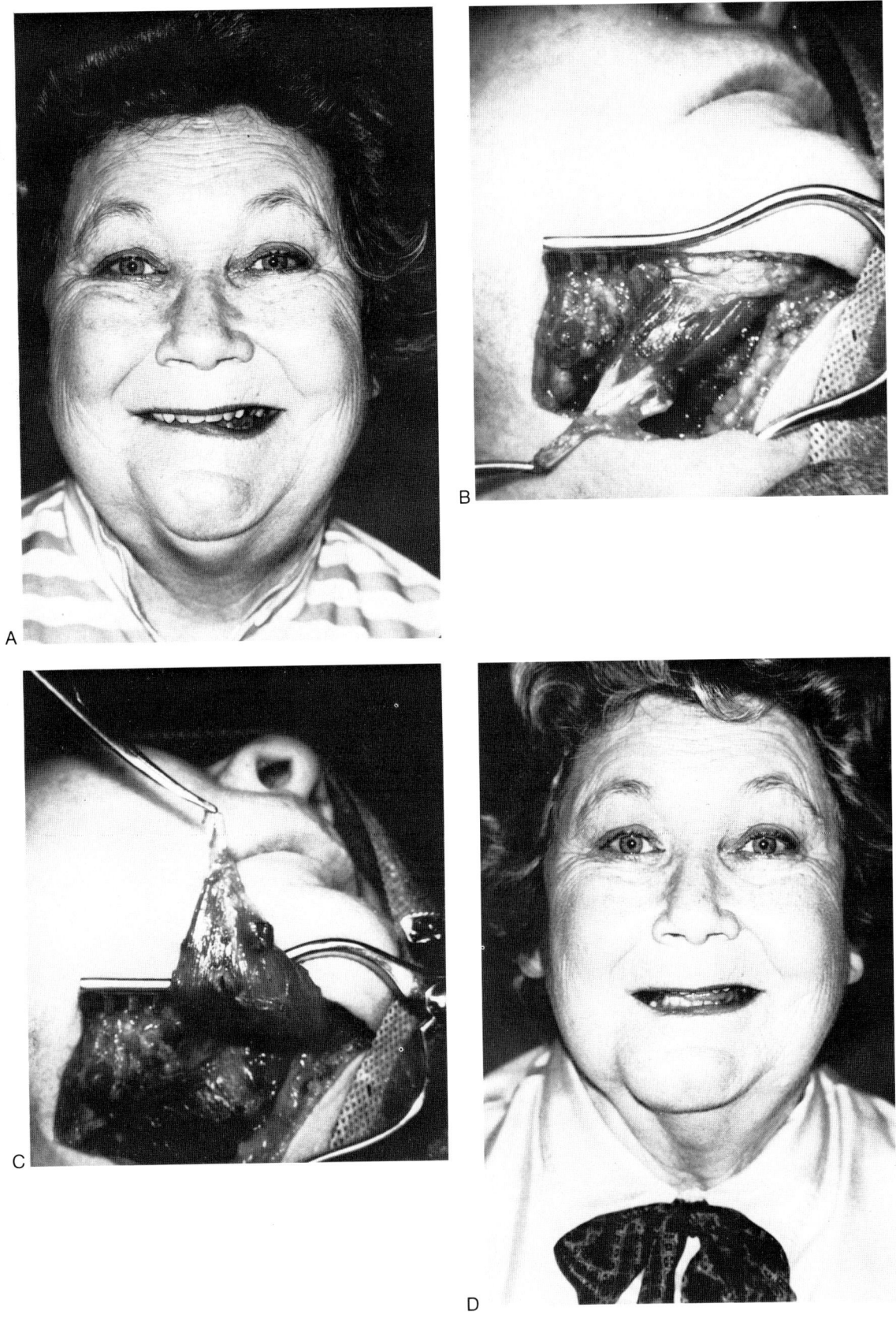

Figure 81. A, Paresis of marginal branch of facial nerve secondary to previous parotidectomy on right side by another surgeon. Note upward pull of right lower lip. B, Anterior belly of digastric muscle isolated and divided at conjoined tendon. C, Conjoined tendon divided into three segments tunneled under skin of chin and sutured into right lower lip. D, Final result, six months postoperative.

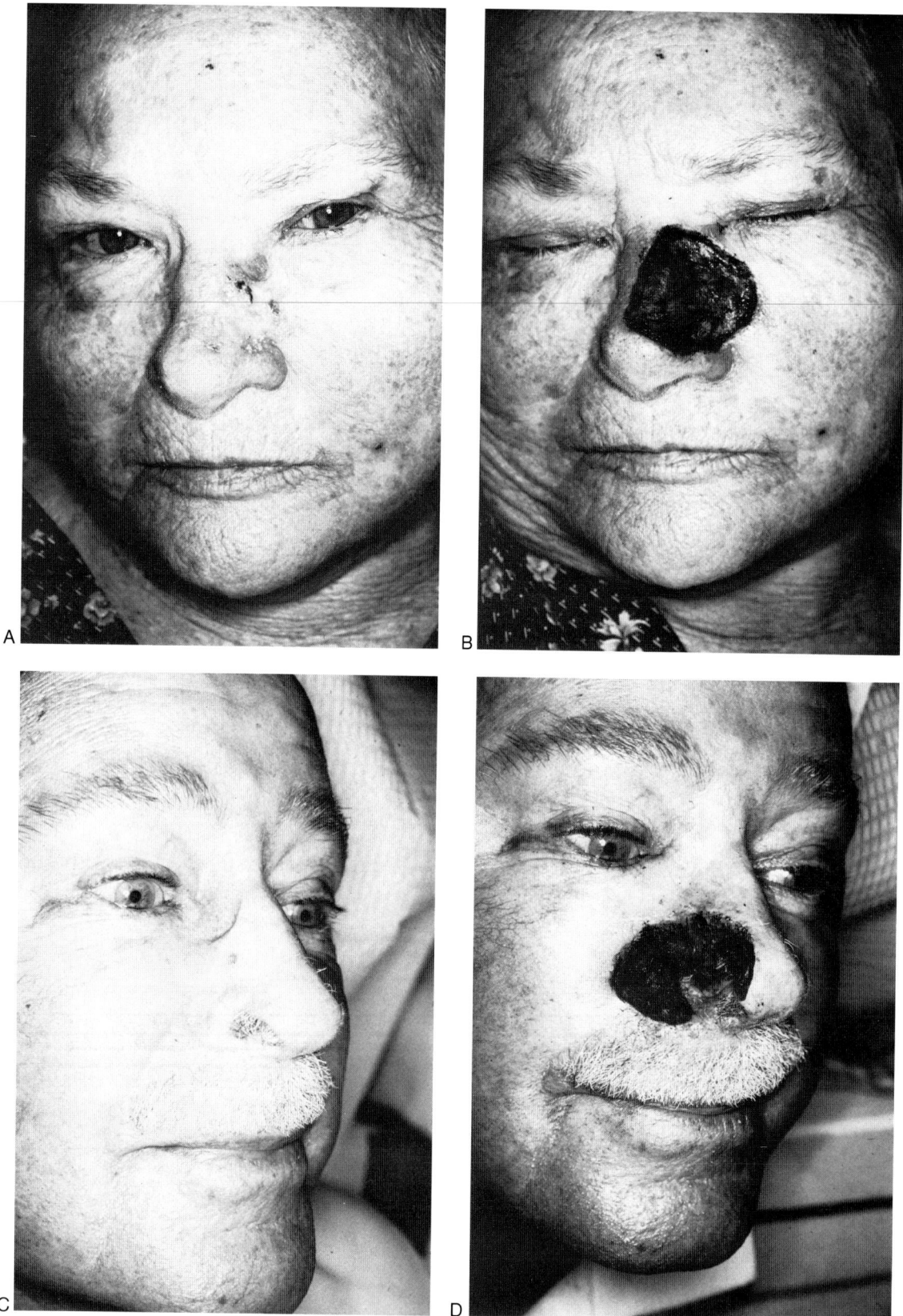

Figure 82. A, Recurrent basal cell carcinoma of left lateral nose. B, Extent of excision by microscopically controlled technique of Mohs' to ensure tumor removal. C, Sclerosing (morphea-form) basal cell carcinoma of left nasal ala. D, Extent of excision by microscopically controlled technique of Mohs' to ensure tumor removal, requiring several stages.

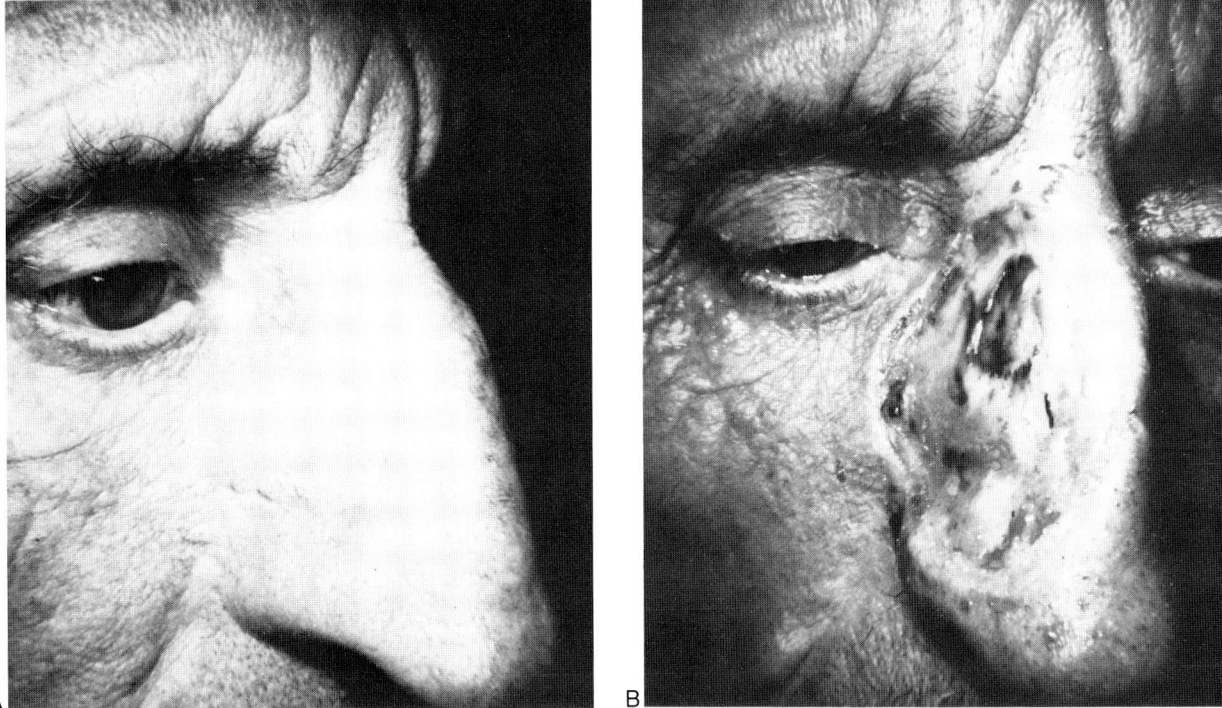

Figure 83. A, Postop status one year. Reconstruction of right lateral nasal defect with nasolabial flap, recurrent basal cell carcinoma in edges of flap. B, Extent of excision necessary to ensure tumor removal by another chemosurgeon.

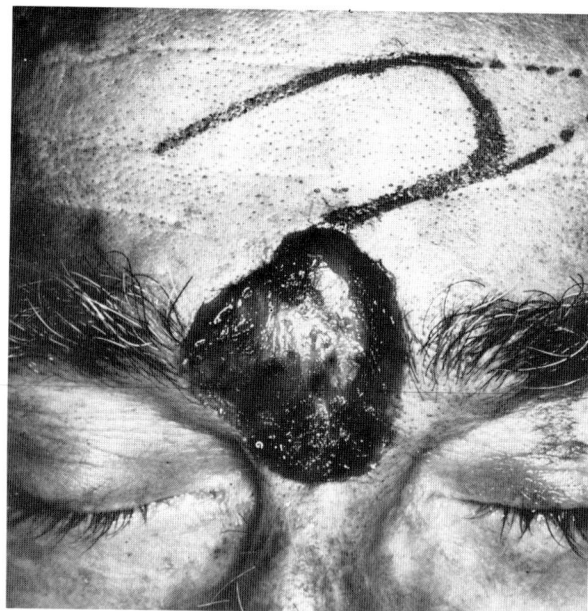
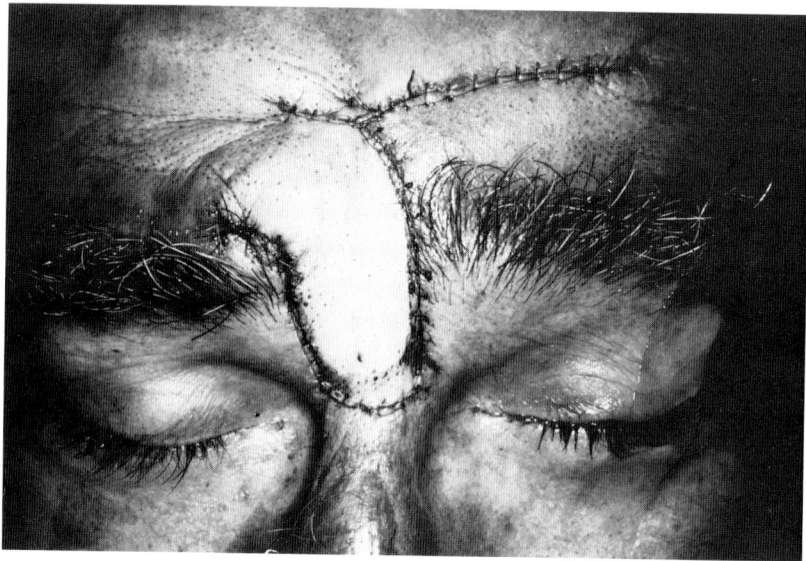

Figure 84. A, Defect resulting in excision of squamous cell carcinoma with forehead flap outlined in immunocompromised patient. B, Final closure.

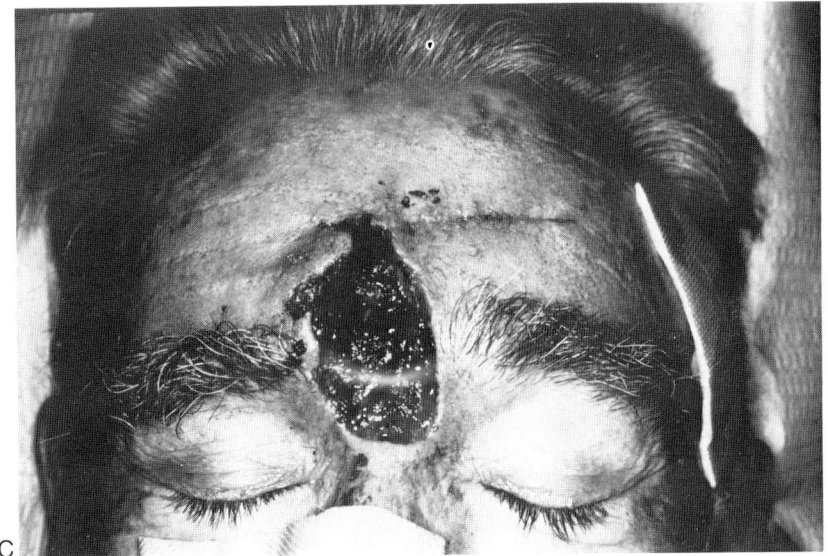

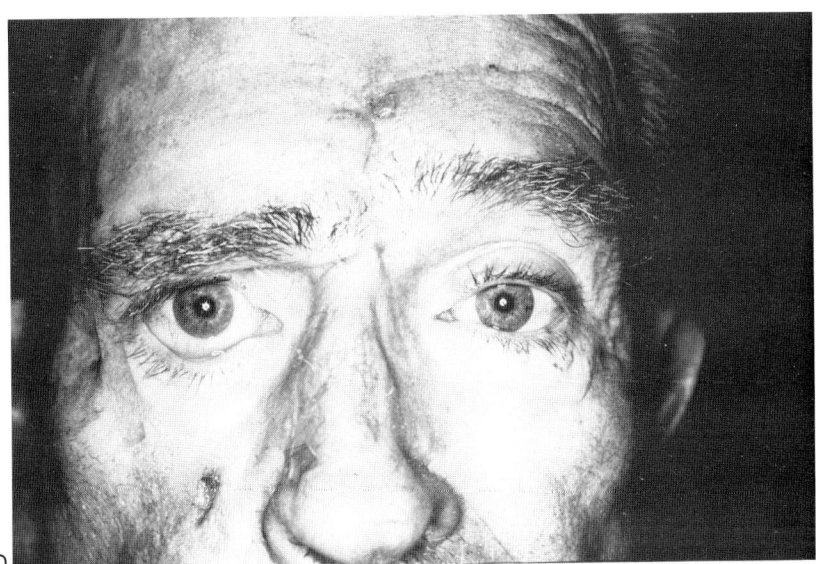

Figure 84. (cont.) C, Complete necrosis of flap. D, Result, four months postoperative with spontaneous healing.

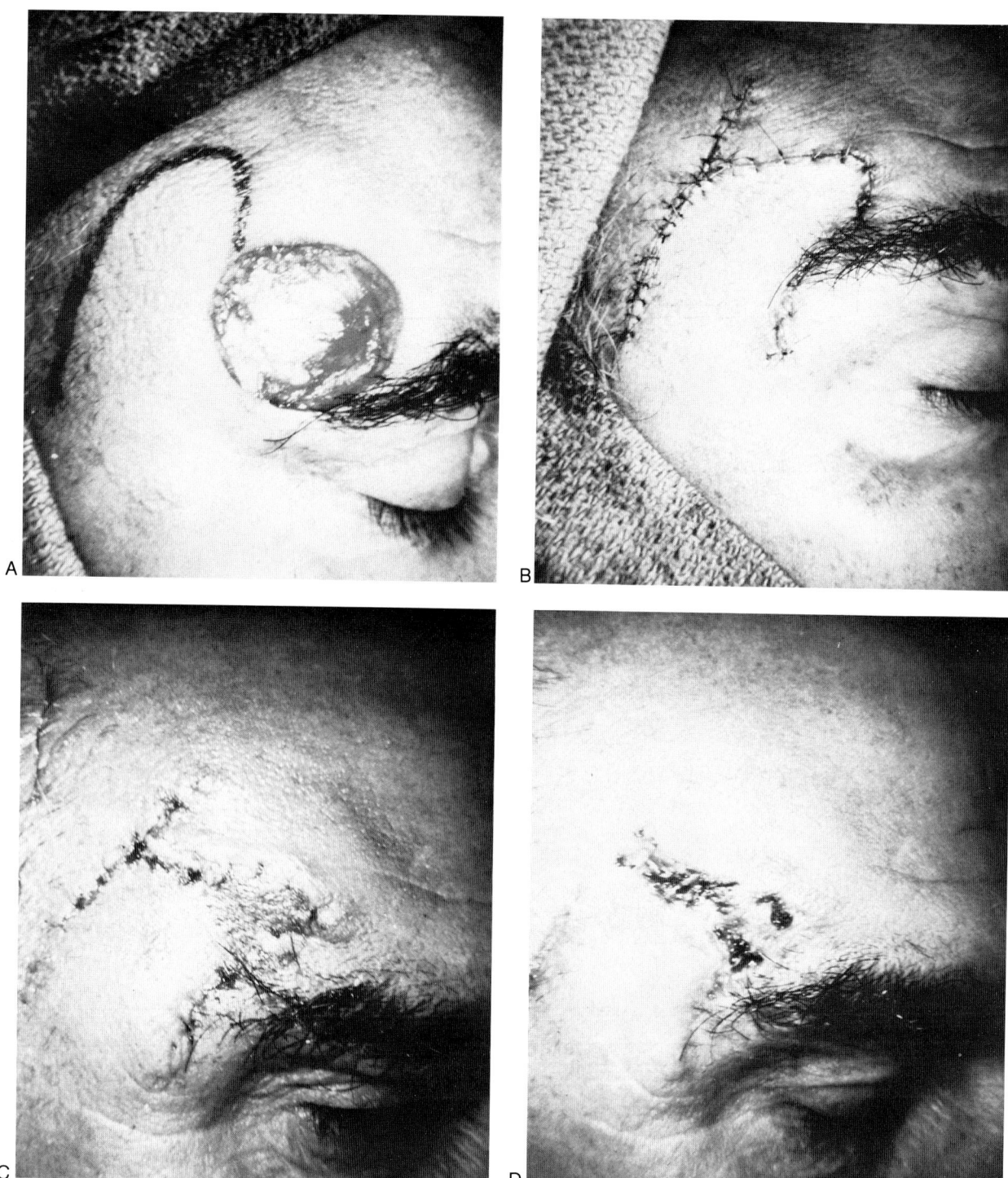

Figure 85. A, Transposition flap outlined for reconstruction of temple defect by another surgeon. B, Final closure. C, One week postoperative, ischemia of tip of flap. D, Three weeks postoperative, necrosis of tip. Note: This flap procedure looks well designed and executed. Presumably the subdermal plexus was compromised in some way.

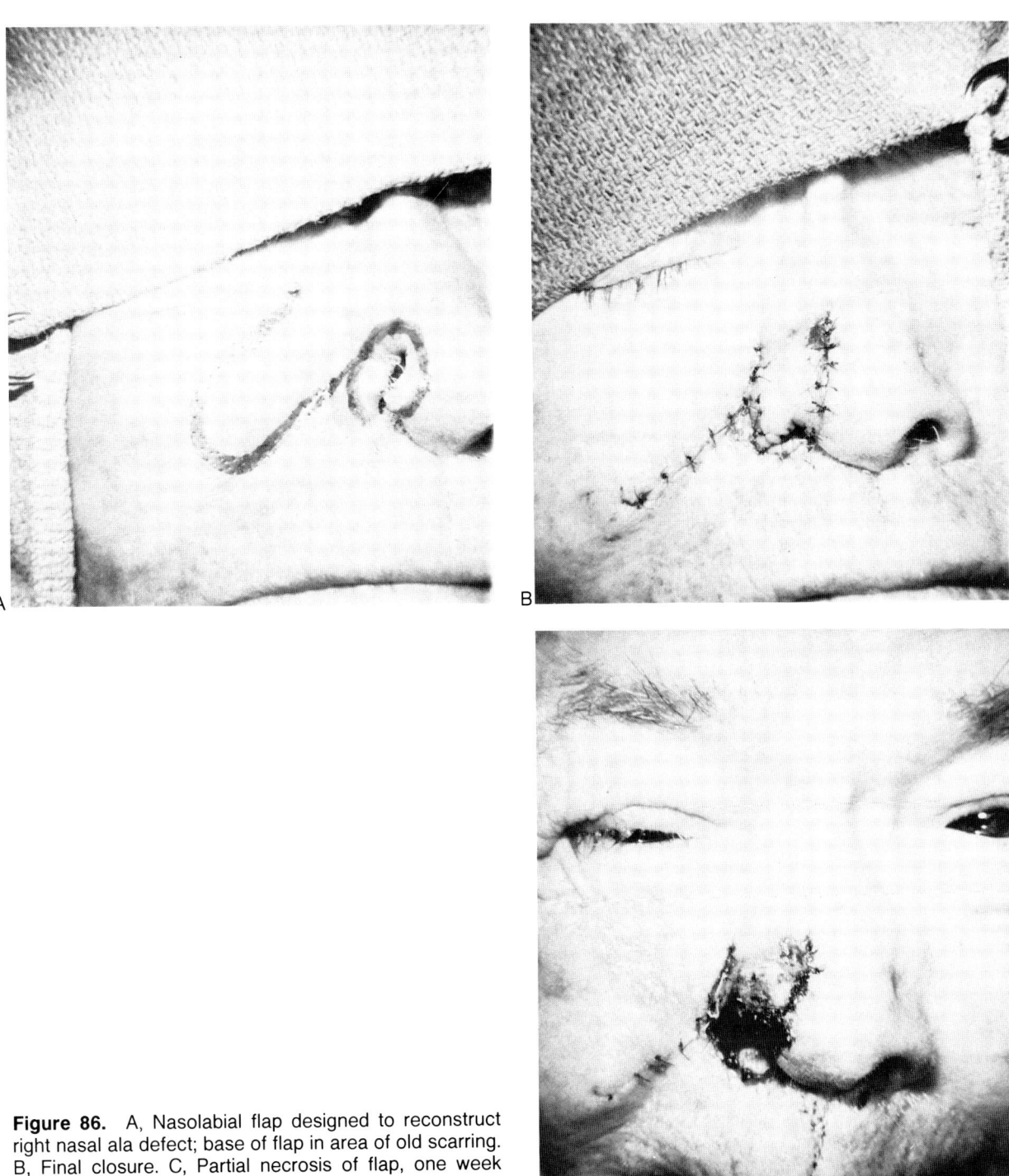

Figure 86. A, Nasolabial flap designed to reconstruct right nasal ala defect; base of flap in area of old scarring. B, Final closure. C, Partial necrosis of flap, one week postoperative. The resulting defect was later reconstructed successfully with a composite auricular graft.

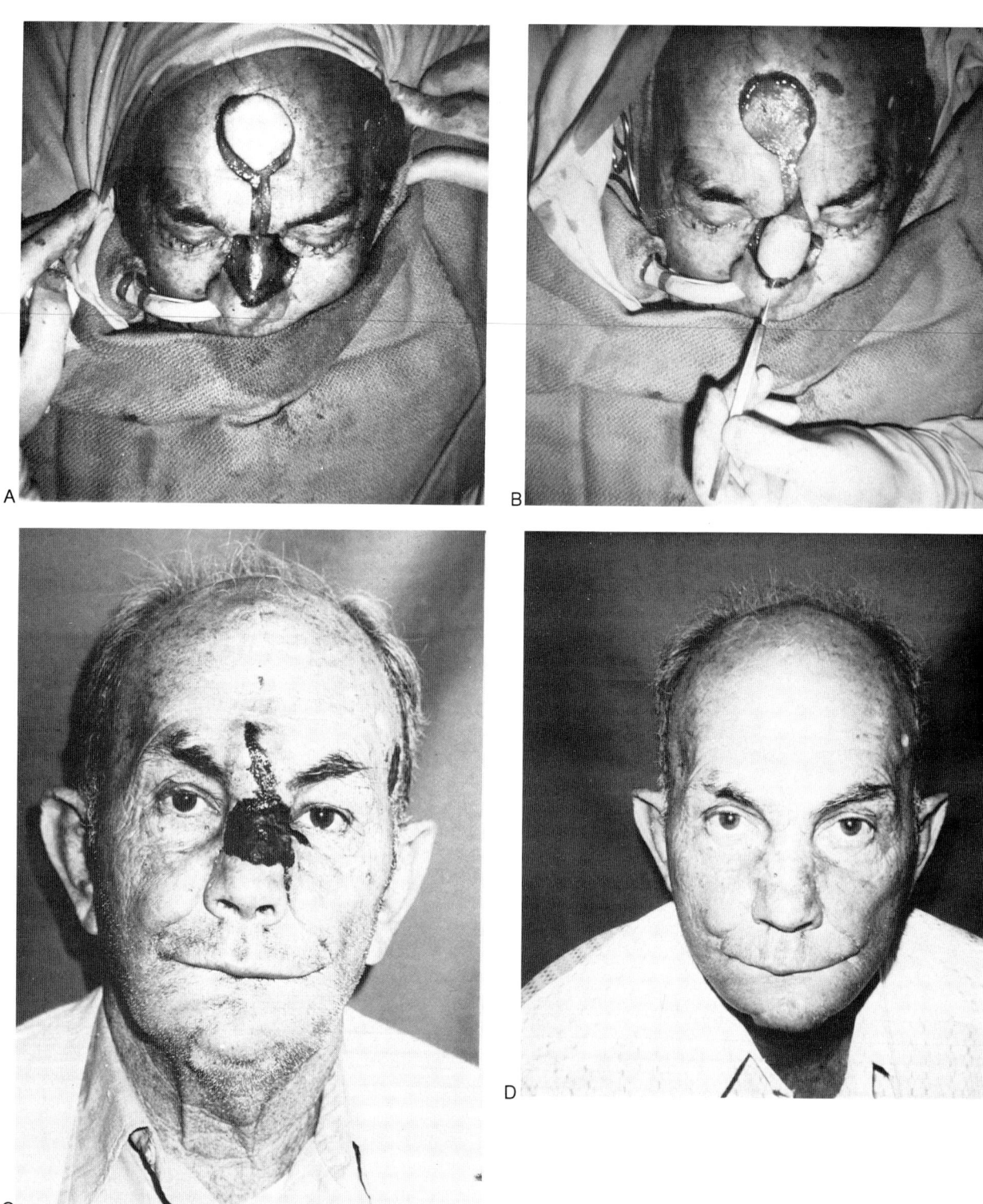

Figure 87. A, Island forehead flap designed for reconstruction of major nasal dorsal defect. B, Flap rotated into place. C, Total flap necrosis. D, Final result following spontaneous healing.

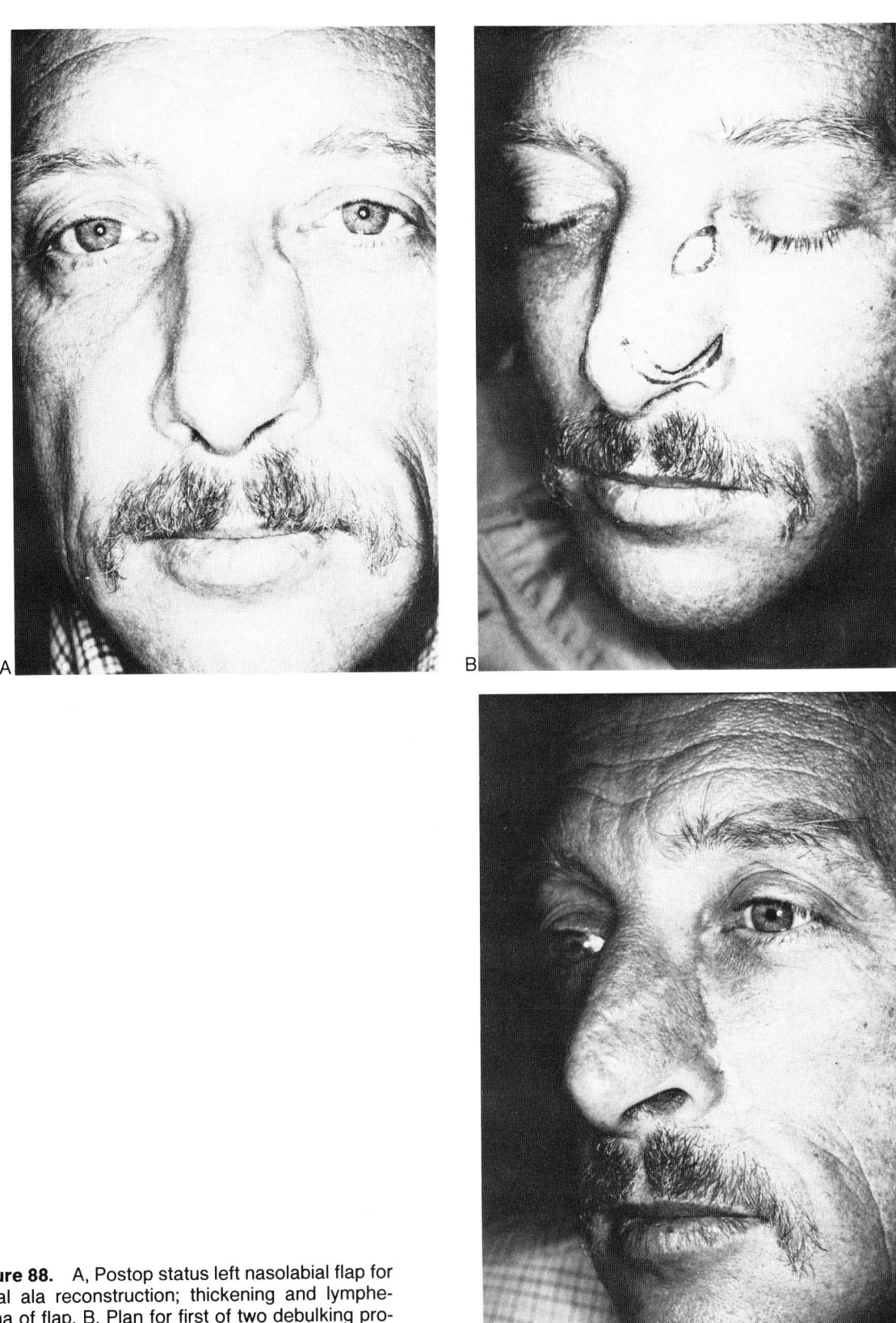

Figure 88. A, Postop status left nasolabial flap for nasal ala reconstruction; thickening and lymphedema of flap. B, Plan for first of two debulking procedures. C, Final result, six months postoperative last procedure.

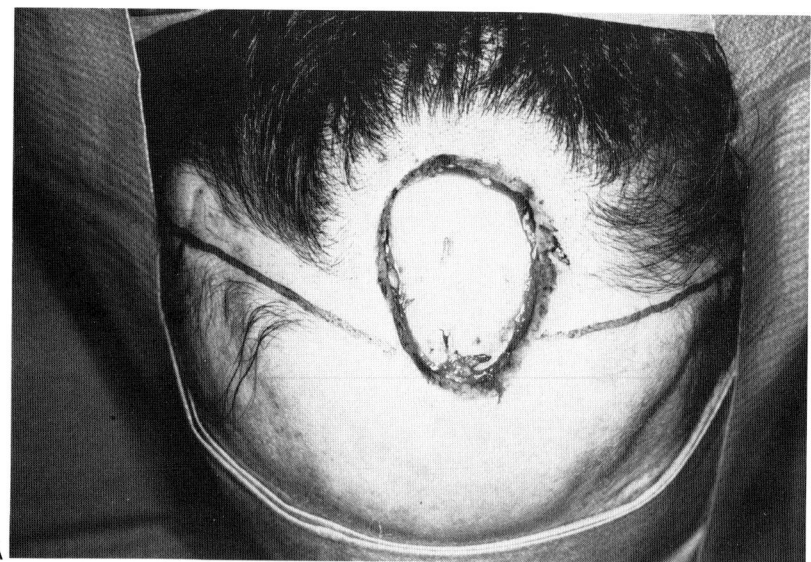
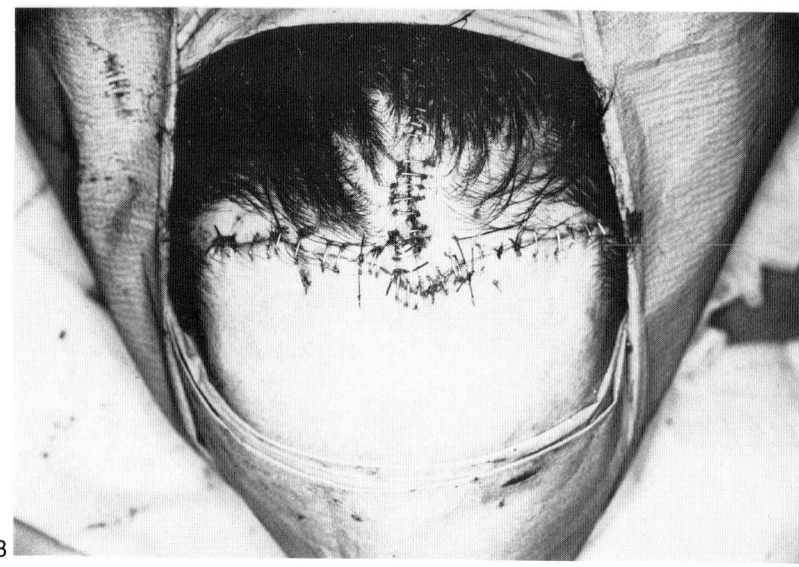

Figure 89. A, Bilateral scalp rotation flaps planned to reconstruct large forehead/scalp defect secondary to excision of extensive recurrent basal cell carcinoma. B, Final closure with tension on edges of wound and tips of flap.

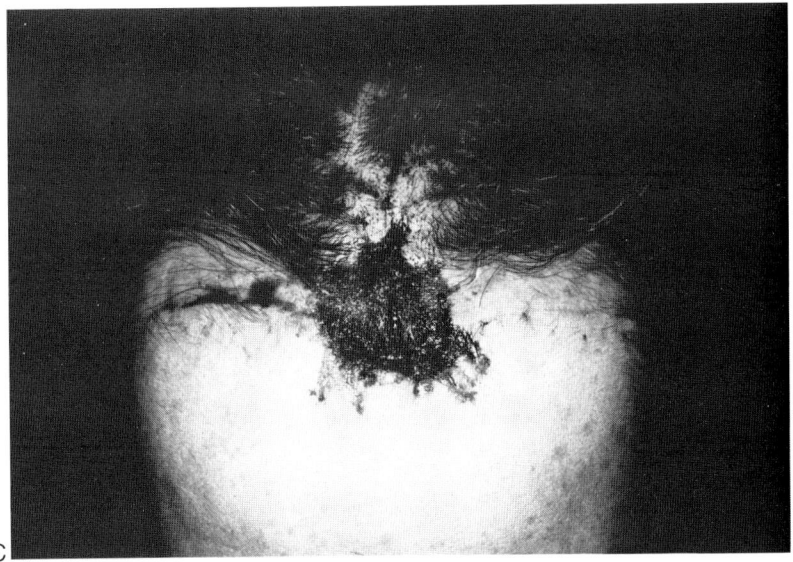
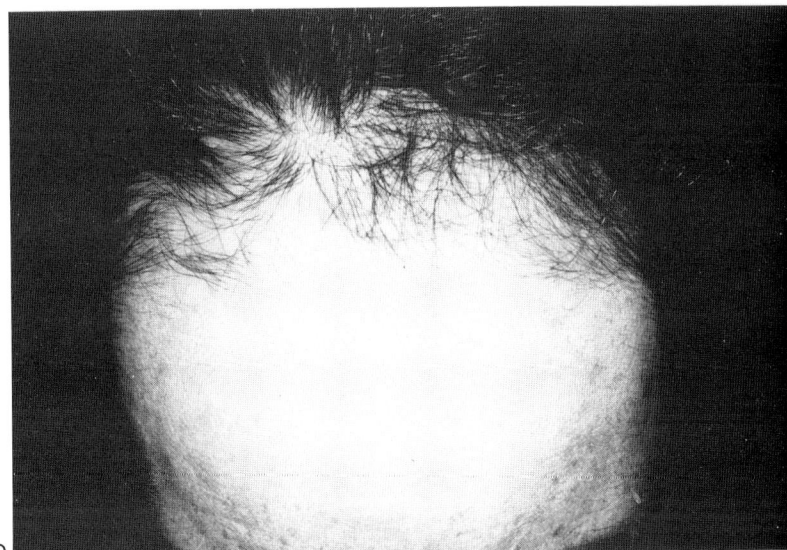

Figure 89. (cont.) C, Partial necrosis of flap tips. D, Final result, two months postoperative.

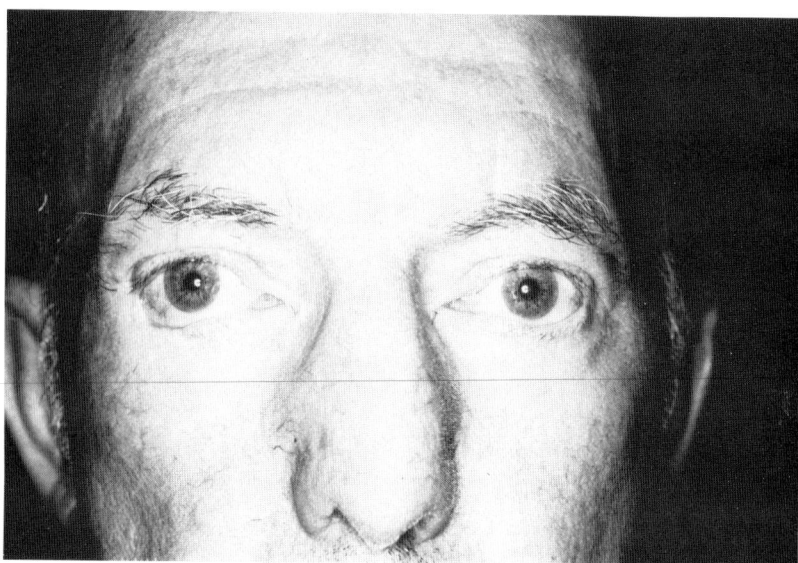

Figure 90. Postoperative status reconstruction of right lower eyelid defect with Mustardé technique by another surgeon, with notch of lower eyelid.

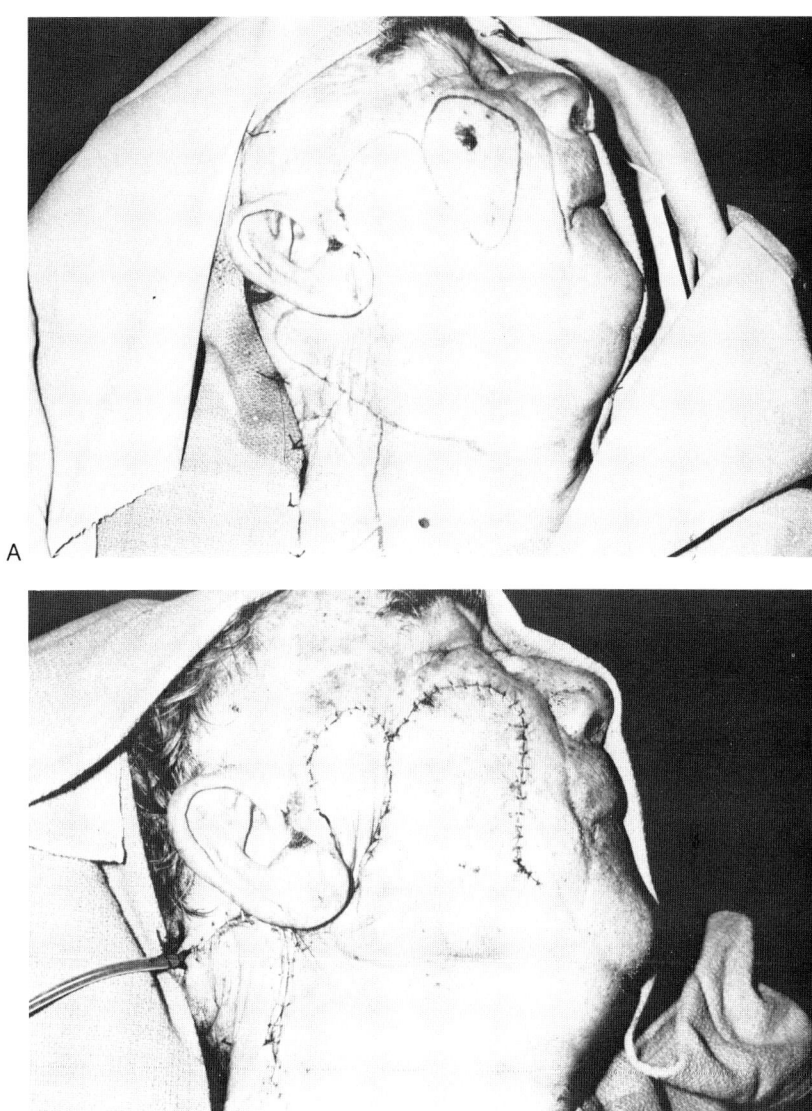

Figure 91. A, Markings for excision of level V nodular melanoma of right cheek prior to wide excision, parotidectomy and radical neck dissection; bilobed cervicofacial flap planned for reconstruction. B, Note compression at base of second lobe.

150 Facial Reconstruction with Local and Regional Flaps

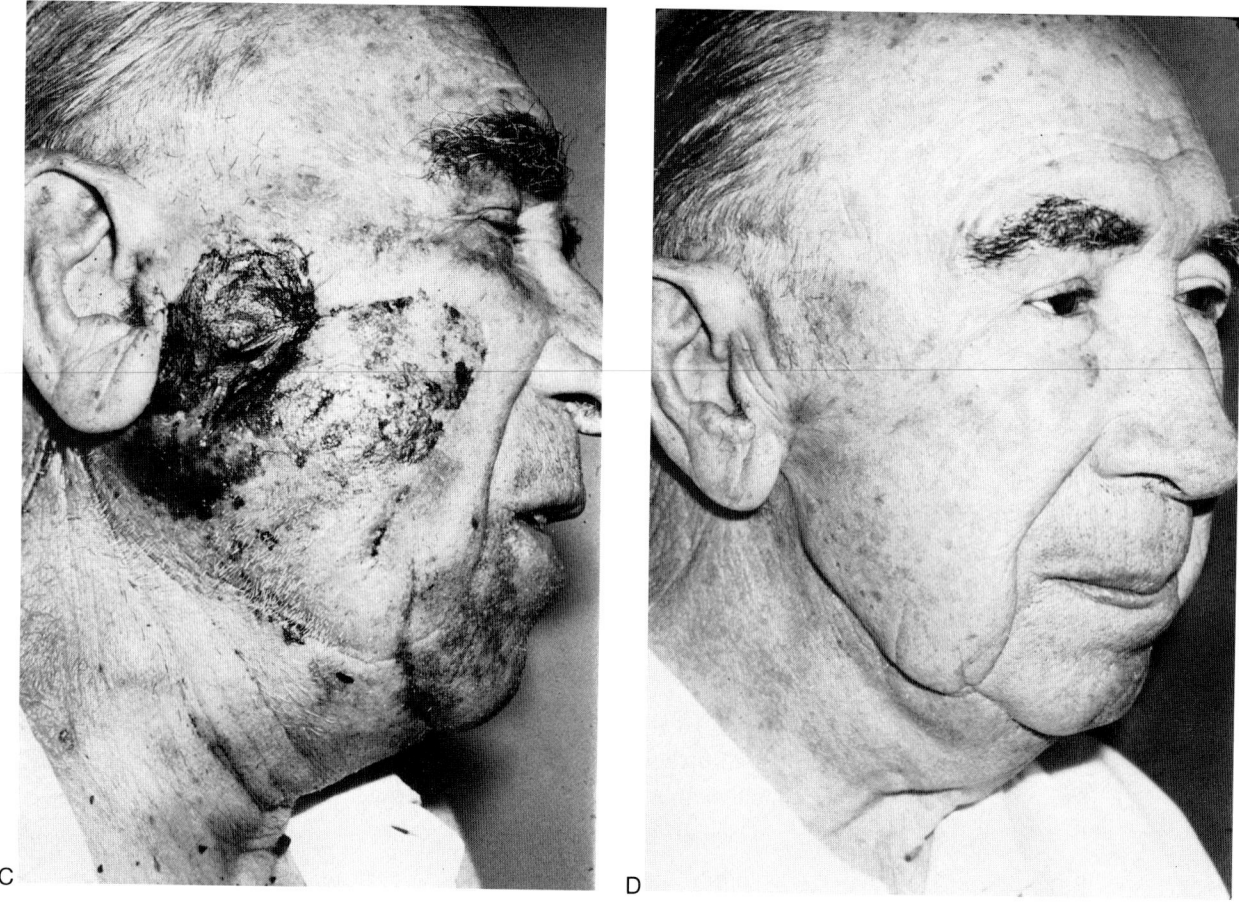

Figure 91. (cont.) C, Necrosis of second lobe of flap. D, Final result, four months postoperative with spontaneous healing.

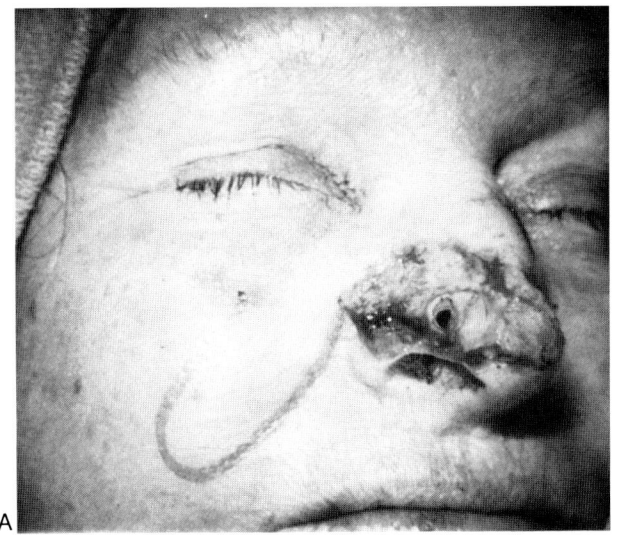
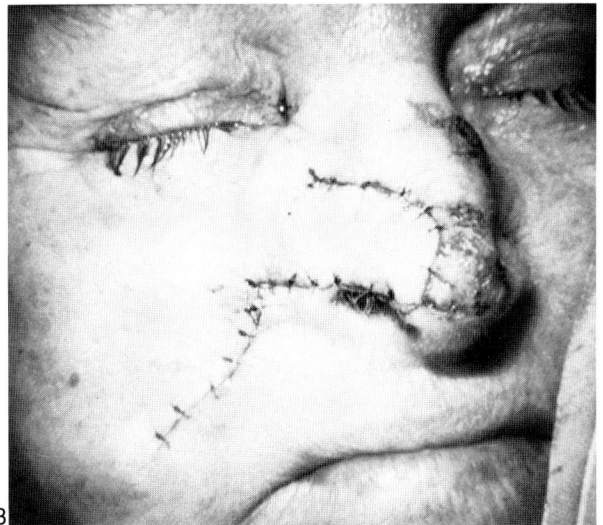
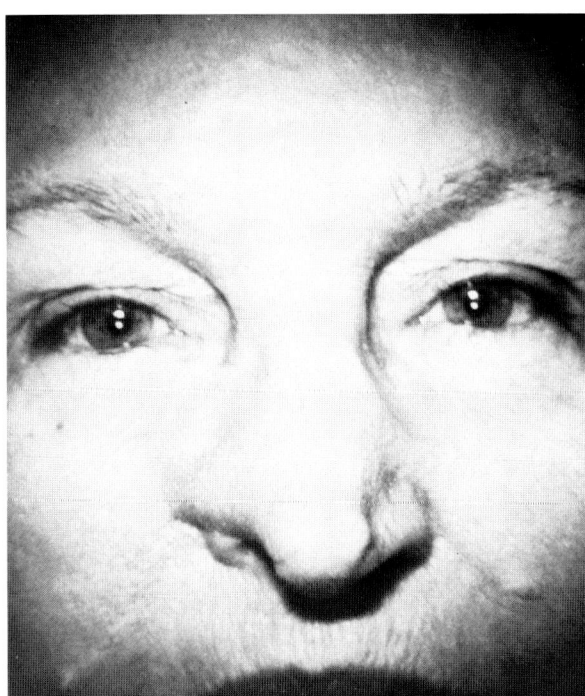

Figure 92. A, Nasolabial flap outlined to reconstruct right nasal ala defect. B, Flap rotated into place was too short and the base of the pedicle was too thick. C, Note thickness of base of pedicle and scarring of nasal tip from secondary healing.

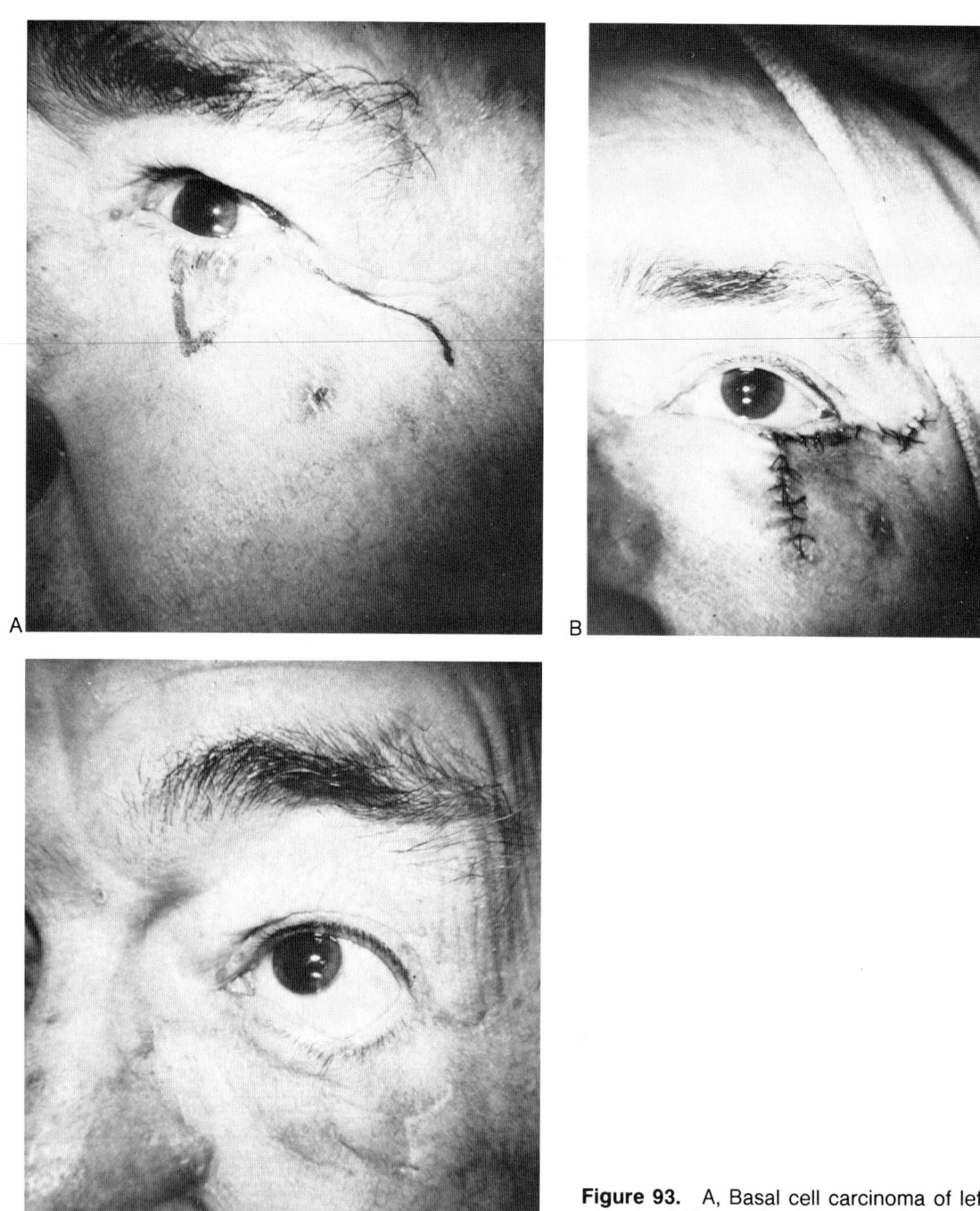

Figure 93. A, Basal cell carcinoma of left lower eyelid with cheek flap outlined, posterior limb of cheek flap was designed too low by another surgeon. B, Final closure. C, Postoperative ectropion development.

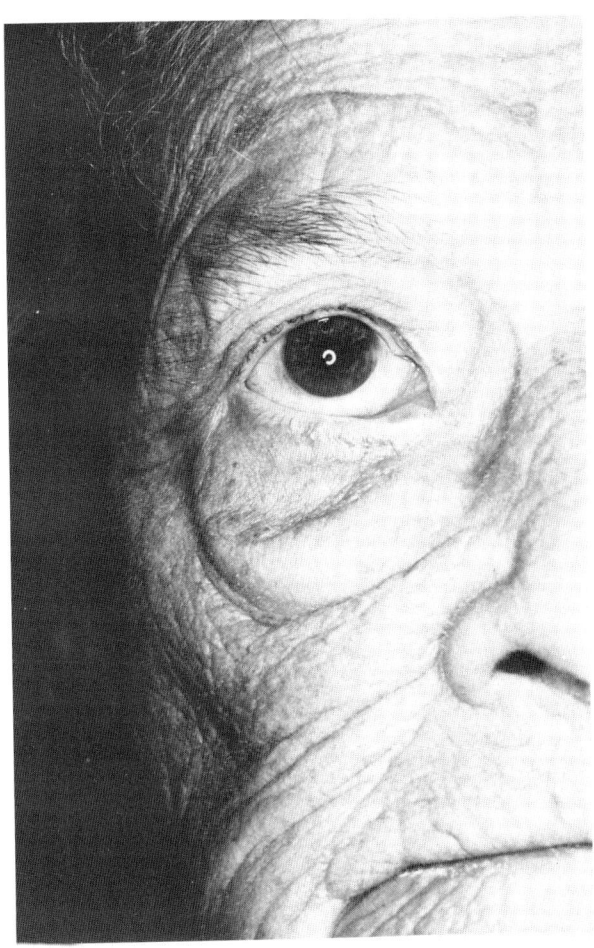

Figure 94. Attempt was made by another surgeon to reconstruct this medial ectropion with a superiorly based nasolabial transposition flap. The patient was left with a deformity on the cheek secondary to the unsuccessful flap, as well as the ectropion.

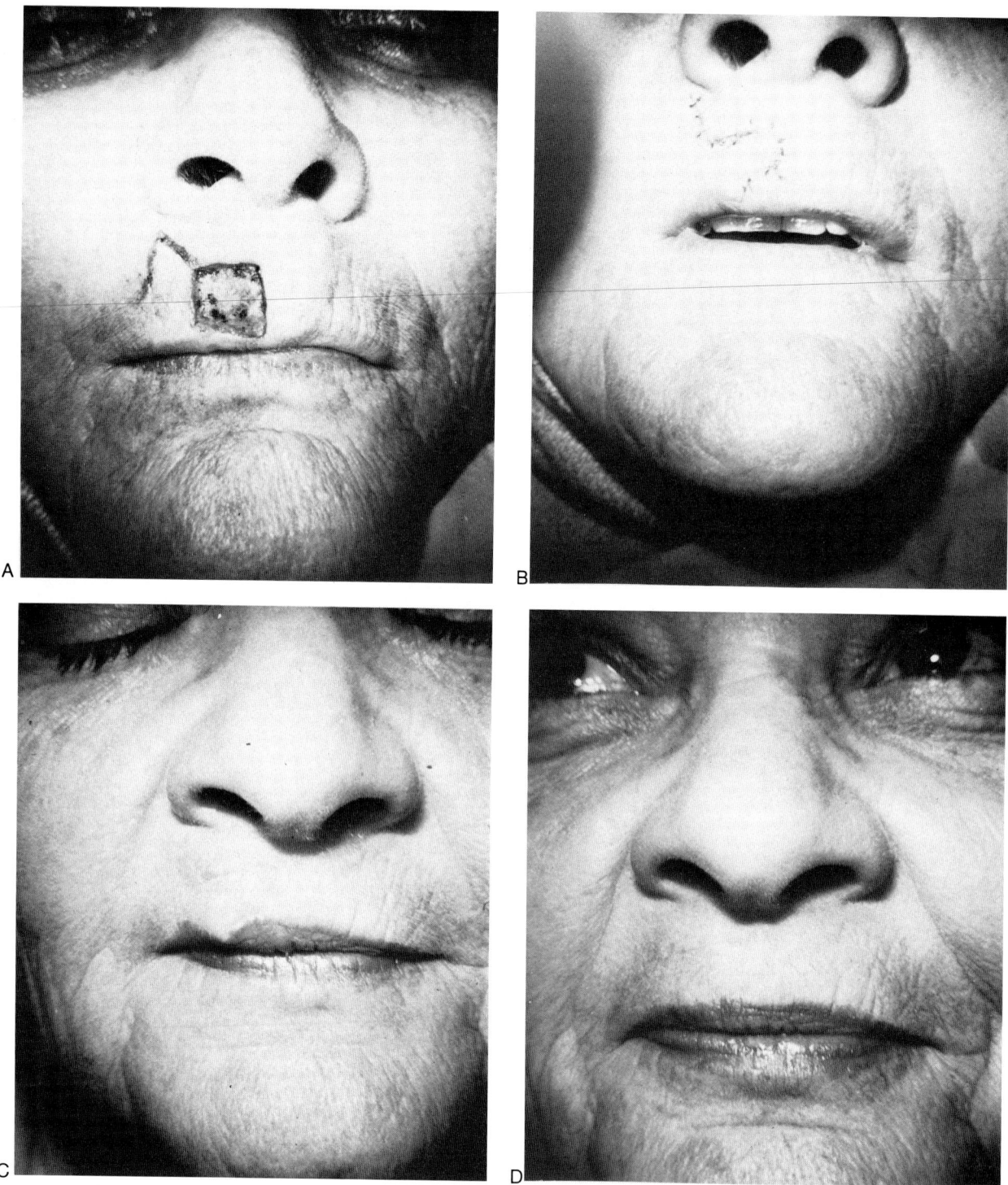

Figure 95. A, Rhombic flap outlined to reconstruct lip defect by another surgeon. B, Rotation point of flap was at the vermilion border. C, Standing cutaneous cone developed at vermilion border. D, Final result after the problem had been corrected by a minor secondary procedure.

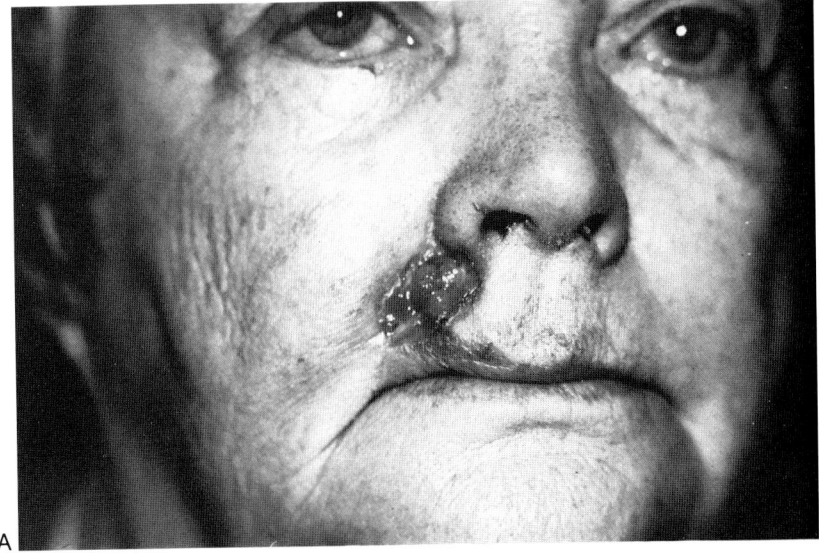
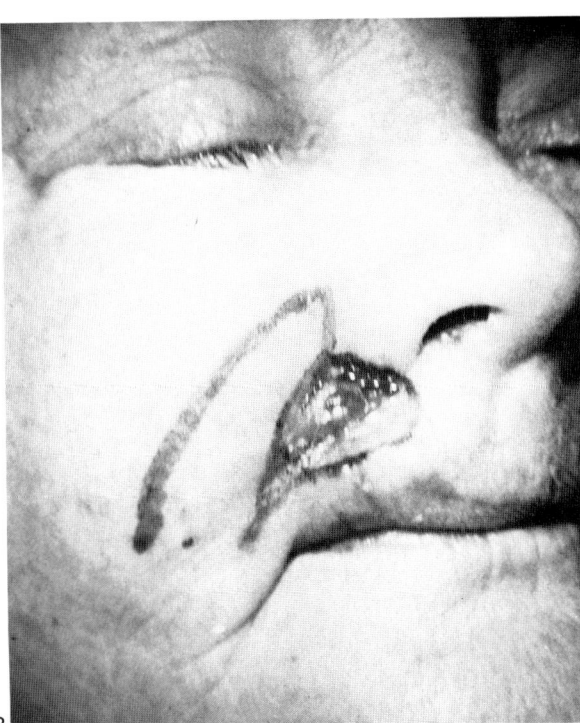

Figure 96. A, Previous excision of basal cell carcinoma of right upper lip with early lip contracture. B, Nasolabial flap outlined by another surgeon to correct this problem. The flap should have been made wide enough to correct the defect and the contracture.

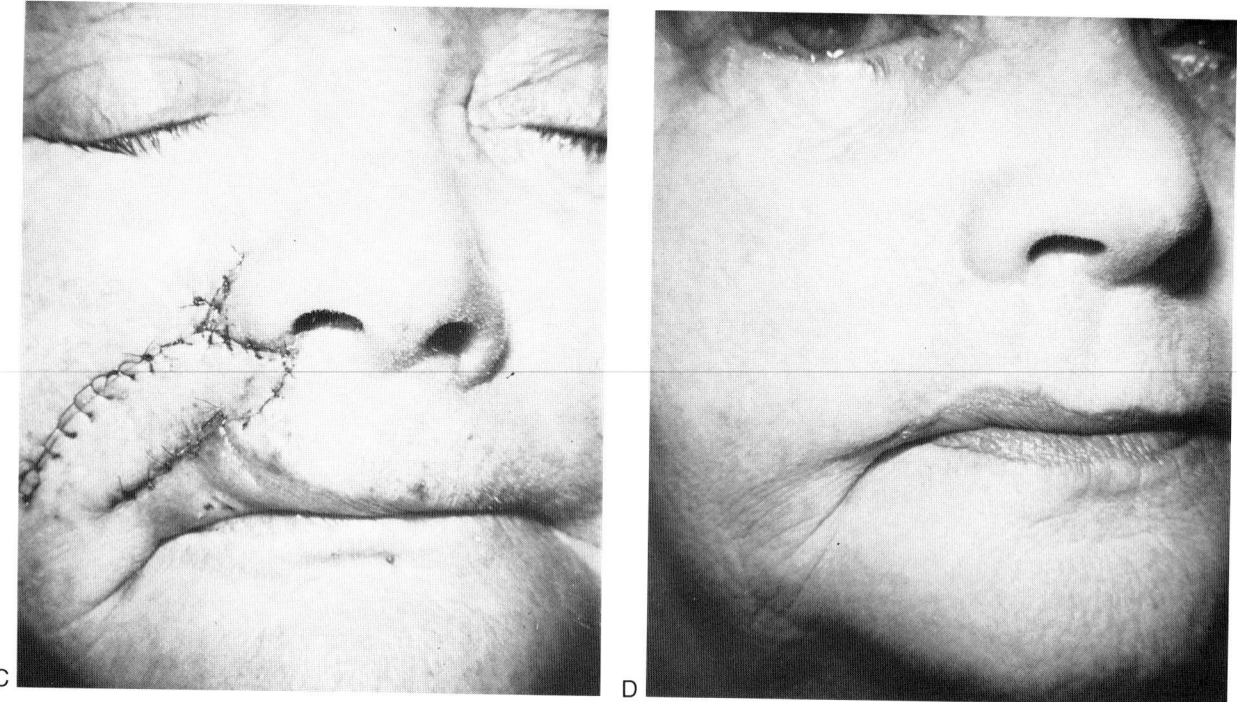

Figure 96. (cont.) C, Defect corrected; contracture is still present. D, Final result with mild contracture of the lip, six months postoperative.

Index

Abbé-Estlander flaps, 62
Advancement cheek flaps, 1, 7, 21, 23
Axial pattern flaps, 1, 2

Bilateral nasolabial flaps, 107
Bilobed flaps, 55
   figures, 56–59
   "pincushioning effect," 55, 58
   primary lobe, 55
   Zimmany's report, 55
Biological problems of patient, 129–130
Blood supply problems, 130

Cervicofacial flaps, 22, 27, 30, 33
   anteriorly-based cervicofacial flaps, 22
   posteriorly-based cervicofacial flaps, 22, 28–29
Cheek flaps
   adjacent, 62
   advancement, 21, 23
   inferiorly-based cheek flaps, 21–22, 24
   rotation cheek flaps, 2, 25, 26
Complications, facial flaps, 127–156
   biological problems, patient, 129–130
   bleeding, 128
   blood supply problems, 130
   complications unique to flaps, 130–131
   failure to control tumor, 128–129
   figures, 132–156
   gravity, 131
   hematologic diseases, 129
   immunologic diseases, 129
   infection, 127–128
   injury to normal uninvolved structure, 129
   lymphedema and thickening, 130
   mechanical factors, 130–131
   Mohs' technique, 129
   planning and design problems, 131
   radiation-induced problems, 129
   self-induced problems, patient, 130
   skin diseases, 129
   stretching of a flap, 130
   surgical complications, 127–130
   systemic diseases, 129
Compound flaps, 1

Dorsal nasal flaps, 37–38, 42–43
Dufourmentel modification, 45, 53

Entropion, 82
   cicatricial, 84–85
Eyelid reconstruction, 79–93
   anatomy, 79
   compared with lip reconstruction, 79
   eyelid defects, 79
   figures, 83–93
   flap reconstruction of eyelid defects involving skin and muscle, 79–80
   flap reconstruction of full thickness eyelid defects, 80
   Hughes technique, 81–82
   medial canthal defects, 82
   Mustardé technique, 80–81
   surgical procedures, 79

Facial flaps, classification of, 1
   according to blood supply, 1
   according to design and execution, 1
   according to tissues composing facial flaps, 1
Forehead flaps, 95–105
   figures, 98–105
   historical background, 95
   horizontal forehead flap, 95
   island forehead flap, 96–97
   midline forehead flap, 95
   technique, 95–96

Glabellar flaps, 37, 39, 40–41
   median, 37
   transposition, 37
   V-to-Y flap, 37

Hematologic diseases, complications, 129
Hughes technique, 81–82
   entropion, 82
   trichiasis, 82

Immunologic diseases, complications, 129
Innervated musculocutaneous lip flaps, 62–63

Interpolation flaps, 1, 6
Island forehead flaps, 96–97

Limberg flap, 45, 47
Lines of maximum extensibility (LME), 45, 49
Lip flaps, 61
77
   Abbé-Estlander flaps, 62
   adjacent cheek flaps, 62
   cupid's bow, 61
   defects greater than one-half lip, 62
   defects less than one-half lip, 61–62
   entire lip involvement, 63
   figures, 64–67
   innervated musculocutaneous lip flaps, 62–63

   orbicularis oris muscle, 61
   thickness of lip, 61
   vermilion border of lip, 61
   W-plasty, 61
Lip reconstruction compared with eyelid reconstruction, 79
Lymphedema and thickening, 130

Medial cantal defects, 82
Midline forehead flaps, 95–96
Multiple flaps facial reconstruction, 107–125
   bilateral nasolabial flaps, 107
   figures, 110–125
   multiple interposition flaps, 107–108
   multiple rotation flaps, 108
   multiple transposition flaps, 107
   multiple Z-plasty, 107
   Mustardé technique, 107
   nasal reconstruction, multiple flaps, 108–109
   serial excision, 108
   upper eyelid tarsoconjunctival flaps, 107
   Z-plasty, 107
Musculocutaneous flaps
   myocutaneous, 98
   skin muscle, 1
Mustardé technique, 80–81, 91, 107

Nasolabial flaps, 9–19
   cutaneous cone, 9, 13
   figures, 11–19
   inferiorly-based nasolabial flaps, 10
   medial cheek tissue, 9
   nasolabial cheek fold, 9
   nasolabial crease, 9
   superiorly-based nasolabial flaps, 9–10
   trapdoor contracture, 10
Nasal reconstruction, multiple flaps, 108–109

Orbicularis oris muscle, 61

"Pincushioning effect", bilobed flaps, 55, 58

Radiation-induced problems, 129
Random pattern flaps, 1, 2
Reconstructive rhinoplasty, Indian method, 95
Relaxed skin tension lines (RSTL), 45, 49
Rhombic flaps, 45–47, 48, 50–52
   Dufourmentel modification, 45, 53
   Limberg flap, 45, 47
   lines of maximum extensibility (LME), 45, 49
   multiple rhomboid flap closures, 45
   relaxed skin tension lines (RSTL), 45, 49
   studies, 46
Rotation flaps, 1, 3
   cheek flaps, 21, 25, 26, 31
   multiple, 108

Serial excision (multiple flaps in sequence), 108
Skin disease, complications, 129
Stretching of a flap, 130
Systemic diseases, complications, 129

Transposition flaps, 1, 4, 5
Trapdoor contracture, 10

Upper lip, 61

Z-plasty, 107